the reverse diabetes diet

control your blood sugar, repair insulin function, & minimise your medication – within weeks

Dr Neal Barnard

This edition first published in 2007 by
Rodale International Ltd
7–10 Chandos Street
London
W1G 9AD

© 2007 Dr Neal Barnard

Published in the US as *Dr Neal Barnard's Program for Reversing Diabetes*

The moral right of Dr Neal Barnard to be identified as the author of this work has been
asserted in accordance with the Copyright, Design and Patents Act of 1988.

Printed and bound in the UK by CPI Bath using acid-free paper from sustainable sources.

1 3 5 7 9 8 6 4 2

A CIP record for this book is available from the British Library

ISBN-13: 978-1-4050-9994-3

This paperback edition distributed to the book trade by Pan Macmillan Ltd

Notice

This book is intended as a reference volume only, not as a medical manual. The information given
here is designed to help you make informed decisions about your health. It is not intended as a
substitute for any treatment that you may have been prescribed by your doctor. If you suspect that
you have a medical problem, we urge you to seek competent medical help. Mention of specific
companies, organizations or authorities in this book does not imply endorsement by the publisher,
nor does mention of specific companies, organizations or authorities in the book imply that they
endorse the book.

   Addresses, websites and telephone numbers given in this book were accurate at the time the book
went to press.

LIVE YOUR WHOLE LIFE™

We inspire and enable people to improve their lives and the world around them

*This book is dedicated to my father, Donald M. Barnard, MD,
a kind and wise physician, and to the participants in our research studies.
I am deeply grateful for your important contribution to this work.*

A Note to the Reader

Here are some important tips before you get started:

See your doctor. If you don't already have a good relationship with a health care provider who is knowledgeable about diabetes, you should get one, and should follow his or her advice about diet, medications, and other aspects of your medical care. I suggest you show this book to your care provider, particularly Chapter 14, which includes information specifically for clinicians. Get your health care provider's okay before making any changes to your diet or exercise routine.

Check your blood glucose. If you have diabetes, it is important that you test your blood sugar with a glucose meter. You already know this is important in order to see if your blood glucose is getting too high. But it might surprise you to know that you'll need to be sure your blood glucose isn't getting too low. 'Now, that's impossible,' you might say. 'My blood glucose never gets down to normal, let alone too low.' But if you are using medications to reduce your blood glucose and you are now adding a powerful diet change, the combination can be very strong. Exercise adds even more power. Diet and exercise alone do not cause blood sugar to get too low, but when they are combined with certain drugs – particularly insulin or drugs that cause your body to release insulin, your blood glucose can drop to very low levels. Your health care provider may need to reduce or eliminate some of your medications. The good news is that this is a sign that your sensitivity to insulin is improving. But you need to be safe. So be sure to use a meter, follow your doctor's advice about testing, and keep your doctor posted on your readings. Read Chapter 7 for more details before you make any diet changes.

Get complete nutrition. Any time you make a diet change, you'll want to make sure you're getting all the nutrients you need. The diet presented in this book is, overall, much more nutritious than other diets. But even so, you'll want to take a few steps to be sure you're not missing anything. You should take a daily multiple vitamin, which will provide vitamin B12, which is not otherwise plentiful in healthy foods, and will easily cover you for all the other vitamins, too.

CONTENTS

PART 3. COMPLETE HEALTH

ACKNOWLEDGEMENTS

The research that culminated in this book was a team effort. I want to express my deepest appreciation to the research volunteers who put up with many early mornings, late nights and needles in performing an important public service. You have taught me a great deal and helped this project immeasurably.

I greatly appreciate the support of the National Institute of Diabetes and Digestive and Kidney Diseases of the National Institutes of Health, particularly Sanford Garfield, PhD, and of the Diabetes Action Education and Research Foundation and its director, Pat DeVoe, RN, BSN, without which this research would not have been possible. Thank you to the American Diabetes Association for the opportunity to share our findings along the way.

Joshua Cohen, MD, of the division of endocrinology at George Washington University, was instrumental in planning and guiding our research work. David J. A. Jenkins, MD, PhD, DSc, of the University of Toronto, is an extraordinary mentor whose generosity with his time, knowledge and ideas is something I hope to pass on to other investigators.

Gabrielle Turner-McGrievy, MS, RD, and Lisa Gloede, RD, CDE, helped extensively in research planning and in guiding our participants towards more healthy ways of eating. Brent Jaster, MD; Amber A. Green, RD; Kim Seidl, MS, RD; Susan Levin, MS, RD; Trulie Ankerberg-Nobis, RD; Dulcie Ward, RD; Jennifer Reilly, RD; and Mary Ellen Wolfe, RN CDE, shared their expertise and guidance with me and our research participants. Robyn Webb and Isabel Clark inspired us all with their culinary wisdom. Thanks to Paul Poppen, PhD, for his expert assistance in planning and executing the statistical analyses. Andrew Nicholson, MD, and Mark Sklar, MD, guided our initial research on diabetes, and Larry Kushi, PhD, provided thoughtful advice along the way. John A. McDougall, MD, and Mary McDougall provided educational materials and wonderful recipes. Jennie Brand-Miller, PhD, of the University of Sydney, kindly answered many questions about her studies of the glycaemic index and its use in clinical practice.

Stanley Talpers, MD, kept a watchful eye on medical issues for our participants, and Brad Moore, MD, served as our safety officer. Thanks to Tara Nicotra, Beatrice Huang, Melinda Beard and Walter Gayle for tackling all the day-to-day issues and keeping our research on track.

Thanks also to Cyril Kendall, PhD; Benoit Lamarche, PhD; and Gary Bradwin for their expertise with laboratory analyses. Special thanks to Ernest P. Noble, MD, PhD, and Terry Ritchie, PhD, of the University of California, Los Angeles, for their generosity and expertise in genetic analyses. Thank you to Donald S. Karcher, MD; Terry Costa; Luce Merino; Estela Day; Patrice Moore; and everyone at George Washington University clinical laboratory client services.

Cael Croft provided the wonderful medical illustrations in this book. I am also very grateful to many individuals who made thoughtful comments on the manuscript, especially Caroline Trapp, APRN, BC-ADM, CDE; Steve Sawmelle; Doug Hall; Stephen Kane; Francelle Wax; Kathy Glissen; Jonathan Balcombe, PhD; Dan Kinburn; Jenn Kaplan; and Benjamin Zoll. Thank you to Lorin O'Toole for critiquing the manuscript and helping with the recipes.

Finally, and especially, thank you to Mary Ann Naples for endless creativity, enthusiasm and wise counsel; Susan Berg, my editor at Rodale, for helping to shape this book into its current form; and Bryanna Clark Grogan for providing wonderful recipes.

INTRODUCTION
A NEW APPROACH TO DIABETES

This book presents a totally new method for preventing, controlling and reversing diabetes based on important research findings that have emerged in recent years.

In studies by my research team, funded by the US government's National Institutes of Health and the Diabetes Action Research and Education Foundation, along with the work of other researchers, we have completely redesigned the dietary approach to diabetes. If your experience with diabetes has been one of gradually escalating medication doses, ever-increasing weight and increasing worry about the risk of complications, you will learn how to reverse those trends.

We will focus on changes in your menu, not on drugs. Yes, medications often have their role, and I will give you details on how they work so you can understand the ones you or your loved ones may be using now. But I would much rather help you scale back on drugs – or eliminate them entirely. Doing that means rethinking the foods that you eat.

Let me emphasize that you will not need to cut calories, limit carbohydrates or stick to small portions. In fact, you can eat until you are full. If you get hungry between meals, you are free to eat more. What we will zero in on is the *type* of food you eat. That has emerged as the critical factor, as you will soon see.

A NEW IDEA

My father, Dr Donald M. Barnard, spent his entire life treating diabetes. He grew up on a family farm but soon realized that farming was not for him. He decided to go to medical school, and after training at Boston's famed Joslin Clinic, he began work at a busy community hospital. He became known as the diabetes expert for the surrounding area. But he and the other doctors – and their patients – often found diabetes puzzling and frustrating. He recounted a telling comment made by the clinic's founder, Dr Elliott P. Joslin, about diabetes research: 'Gentlemen, we don't need a big research grant. What we need is a new idea.'

Dr Joslin made that observation back in the 1950s, and the need has only grown more urgent as the incidence of the disease has exploded. Worldwide, about 200 million people are living with diabetes.[1] Until now, most have found the condition to be at best an exercise in drudgery. With daily blood tests and medications that promise only to slow the disease's inevitable damage, a patient's life becomes a waiting game, with one complication arising after another – from nerve symptoms to visual changes and heart and kidney problems.

Now, at last, we're on the cusp of real change. I'm talking not just about a bold new idea, but about an entirely new approach to diabetes that has been tested and proven.

In a series of research studies conducted with Georgetown University and George Washington University in Washington, D.C., our research team has proven that many people with diabetes can think beyond delaying inevitable decline and improve their health dramatically. They can cut their blood sugar, increase insulin sensitivity and reduce or eliminate medications, and they can do this with a simple set of diet changes. Unlike with medication treatments, the 'side effects' of the menu change are good ones: weight loss, lower cholesterol levels, lower blood pressure and increased energy.

From the beginning, our studies aimed higher and took a more aggressive approach to diabetes than clinicians had in the past. The first study was small – just 13 patients – and it tested a programme that relied entirely on changes in diet. There was no new drug, no magical supplement – not even an exercise programme. But the results were amazing. Two-thirds of patients improved so much that they were able to reduce or eliminate their medications within 12 weeks. The study was published in *Preventive Medicine* in 1999.[2]

Then, in a second study, this one involving 59 patients with varying degrees of blood sugar control – some healthy, others prediabetic or diabetic – we studied *why* diet change works. It became clear that the diet shift actually caused a fundamental change in the body itself. In 14 weeks, the diet led to a 24 per cent improvement in insulin sensitivity – that is, the body's ability to respond to insulin, the sugar-storing hormone that is dysfunctional in diabetes. Participants whose blood sugar levels were in the abnormal range saw them promptly return to where they belonged. While exercise could increase the benefits even further, *diet changes alone* were powerful enough to boost insulin sensitivity and bring blood sugar under better control. The results were presented at the American Diabetes Association Scientific Meeting in 2004 and were published in the *American Journal of Medicine* in 2005.[3]

These studies suggest that this new approach may be the most powerful nutritional plan ever devised for diabetes. We can do more than try to *compensate* for malfunctioning insulin, as doctors have done for decades with various medications. Rather, we can help the body's own insulin work properly again by directly addressing – and improving – the cells' sensitivity to it, which is the key issue in type 2 diabetes. Even when the disease has evolved to the point of serious complications, it is not too late for marked improvements to occur.

Starting in 2003, with the support of the National Institutes of Health, we conducted a new research trial to compare our diet with the gold standard: the American Diabetes Association (ADA) guidelines. These guidelines are sensible and well established. Millions of people in the US follow them and use the exchange lists, as well as cookbooks developed from the guidelines, to manage the disease. But all too often, a familiar story ensues: despite everyone's best efforts, the disease worsens over time. Our goal was to see if we could improve things. The study was conducted with George Washington University and the University of Toronto and included 99 individuals with type 2 diabetes. The participants were randomly assigned to either a standard diabetic diet based on the ADA guidelines or to the more aggressive diet you will learn about shortly.

In a careful analysis that kept exercise and medication use constant, we found that the new diet controls blood sugar three times more effectively than the previous 'best' diet. It also accelerates weight loss and controls cholesterol better than the old gold standard. Other investigators have shown that this kind of diet also has dramatic benefits for the heart and leads to a healthy drop in blood pressure. It allows many individuals to take charge of their lives again and to return to health and vigour.

This book translates these scientific breakthroughs into tools that you can use, including an easy-to-follow plan with simple diet guidelines, menus and recipes.

A NEW UNDERSTANDING OF TYPE 1 DIABETES

Type 1 diabetes is much less common than type 2. It is usually diag-nosed in childhood and is invariably treated with insulin – hence its former names, childhood-onset diabetes and insulin-dependent diabetes.

Unlike people with type 2 diabetes, those with type 1 always need to take insulin. But they can use diet and lifestyle changes to keep doses to a minimum and reduce the risk of complications. We also have a new – and surprising – understanding of the *fundamental causes* of type 1 diabetes. It may surprise you to learn that the process that leads to type 1 diabetes begins when the body's immune system attacks the insulin-producing cells of the pancreas. As you will see, new research has revealed what appears to spark this attack and what can help to prevent it.

PERSONAL SUCCESS

Let's take a look at the experiences of real people who followed the programme described in this book.

Nancy

Nancy learned about our research study from an advertisement in a newspaper. She had been diagnosed with type 2 diabetes 8 years earlier. A cousin of hers had lost some of his eyesight to the disease, and failed kidneys left him on dialysis. Nancy did not want that to be her future. She was going to fight back.

Before she joined our study, things had been going in the wrong direction. Although she had followed a diet designed for diabetes, her blood sugar was gradually worsening, and the diet did nothing to stop her weight from creeping upwards.

Two years after her diagnosis, her doctor put her on her first diabe-tes medication. Eventually, he felt she needed two medications. Still her blood glucose level continued to rise. As she entered our study, her HbA1c level – the key index of blood glucose control, which ought to be below 7.0 per cent – was an unhealthy 8.3 per cent.

Nancy joined the study because she liked the focus on food rather than on drugs. With the explosion of diabetes in the population, she intuitively felt that the problem had to be the kinds of food we eat and that the solution had to be there, too.

We showed her how to change her diet. There were no limits on how much she could eat or on how many calories or grams of carbohydrates she could have. But we did ask her to make a major change in the *type* of food she chose.

At first, we also asked her *not* to exercise – that is, not to change her exercise habits – because we wanted to see what diet changes alone could do. That suited her just fine – she was very busy at her office, working long hours every day, and exercise was not exactly her thing. At least not yet.

As she began to follow our recommendations, her weight started to fall, along with her blood glucose, the latter with surprising speed. After years of going up and up and up, the trend started to reverse. After 11 weeks, she stood on the scales: she had lost 6.4 kg (1 st). And when she rolled up her sleeve and we checked her HbA1c, we found that it had dropped from 8.3 per cent to 6.9 per cent. All in about 3 months' time. Her insulin sensitivity was returning.

Nancy's blood sugar continued to fall. In fact, it fell so much that it became clear that her medications were now too strong for her. The combination of the drugs she had been taking, along with the new, powerful diet changes, actually left her blood sugar too low. It was time to reduce her medications. But as we cut back on her doses, it turned out not to be enough. After several more months, we had to stop one of them altogether.

A little more than a year after joining the study, she was 18 kg (2 st 9 lb) lighter. She was on one diabetes medication, not two (it remains to be seen if she can eliminate the second one). And even though she is taking less medication, her HbA1c is better than it was before – 6.8 per cent at her last test.

'The payoff is just incredible,' she said. 'But it's not just the weight loss. My numbers have gotten dramatically better.'

And there was more – another benefit she had not anticipated. For years, she had had arthritis pain so severe she could not open a jar. After a few months of a new diet, she suddenly realized that her arthritis symptoms were completely gone. (There is actually a fascinating body of scientific literature on diet and arthritis, which I summarized in an earlier book, *Foods That Fight Pain*.) The best part of the story: Nancy's experience is not unusual for people who make the diet changes you will read about shortly.

Vance

Vance was just 31 years old when he was diagnosed with diabetes. He had just changed to a new doctor, and the diagnosis came after a routine blood test. Both of his mother's parents had had the disease, but up until that point, Vance had been in more or less good health. He had been a police officer for 12 years and now worked in a bank, and he was not in the habit of calling in sick.

Diabetes changed everything. 'If I didn't lose a leg or go blind, I could end up on dialysis,' he said. And the truth was, he was not in such perfect shape. He had gradually gained weight over the years, and at just under 1.8 m (6 ft) tall, he weighed 124 kg (19 st 7 lb). 'I didn't really take my diet or my health very seriously,' he said. 'I grew up on steak sandwiches, pork chops and chicken. We had some vegetables, but not a lot of fresh foods. I didn't exercise. I just didn't take any of this very seriously.'

Along with weight problems came difficulties with sexual performance. Impotence affects many men with diabetes and is common in men who are overweight. His doctor started him on metformin, a commonly prescribed medication for reducing blood sugar.

Vance learned about our research study and decided to volunteer – despite a few misgivings about the prospect of changing his diet. 'I never had any diet restrictions or rules before,' he said. 'I never tried to control my diet before. I always ate whatever I wanted.' But his wife had been a vegetarian for some time, and she was excited that Vance was ready for a change, too.

The payoff came pretty quickly. His weight started to fall, and over a year's time, he lost – to his surprise – about 27 kg (4 st 3 lb). His HbA1c, which had been 9.5 per cent at the beginning of the study, fell to 7.1 per cent after just 2 months. Fourteen months into the study, it had dropped to 5.3 per cent. His doctor was thrilled and said it was time to stop the metformin.

One more surprise: his problems with sexual performance virtually disappeared within 3 months. 'I haven't been in this good shape since I was in the police academy. It is like a weight has been lifted off of me,' he said. 'When I told my mother what I was doing – that I had changed my diet — she was so happy, she nearly cried, because my dad died at 30. When my grandfather died, I was the oldest male in my immediate family. We tend to check out pretty quick. But she saw I was on a different path. I was taking care of myself.'

TAKING CONTROL

The diet Nancy and Vance embraced — and that I hope you are about to begin — is designed to do much more than simply palliate diabetes, as other diets do. It is designed to tackle the fundamental causes of the disease.

As those who participated in our study learned, blood sugar levels that creep steadily upward can also fall. The road to diabetes is in fact a two-way street.

Whether you have type 2 diabetes and want to gain control of your health or have type 1 diabetes and need to reduce the disease's intrusion on your life, this programme was designed with you in mind.

However, our research — and this book — also targets a broader purpose. More and more people, including a surprising number of children, are diagnosed with diabetes every day. They and their families pay a high personal price for dealing with the condition. And our health services are also struggling to keep up with the costs. For many people at risk, it is simply a matter of time before they are diagnosed. It is our hope that a new direction in diet and nutrition, if applied broadly enough, can go a long way towards solving these problems.

This programme is truly a revolution in the way we think about this otherwise unforgiving disease. Diabetes is no longer a condition you simply have to live with. It need not slowly and inevitably get worse. Quite the opposite. If you have diabetes, it is time for you to get your life back.

We will not cater to your diabetes. Rather, this programme is designed to help you understand the *cause* of diabetes and how to *correct it* to the fullest extent that diet and lifestyle changes possibly can. If you do not have the disease but are at risk, this is a powerful programme for preventing it.

'Is this programme for me?' you may be asking. The answer is an emphatic yes. Here's why.

- **Whether you like to cook or not, you can easily make the diet changes you need.** I make this point because some people imagine that changing their diet means hours of work in their kitchen. If you inwardly groan at that thought, I sympathize: I learned long ago that my temperament is not suited to cooking. Perhaps I was born with the 'room service gene', and maybe you were, too. So I will show you how to plan a healthy menu and how to make it work for you whether or not you like to cook. Many of our research participants travel, eat at restaurants or eat in staff cafeterias. This programme worked for them, and it can work for you.

- **It does not matter whether you love exercise or have never been able to stick with an exercise plan.** The improvements described above were made *without exercise*. In fact, all of our research studies omit exercise because we need to isolate the effect of diet changes in order to put them to a good test. Having said that, exercise is an important part of any diabetes treatment regime, and this book will show you how to bring it into your life in a sensible, safe and effective way. If, however, you are unable to engage in significant exercise because of joint problems, a heart condition or severe obesity, or if you find you're just not able to stick with an exercise programme, you will be glad to know that the benefits of our diet change are not dependent on any alteration of your activity levels.

- **If you have felt that you just cannot stick with a diet, I completely understand.** That's why we will focus solely on *what* you eat, not *how much*. You can eat until you are full and have snacks when you want them. You will have to invest some energy, however: you will have to learn to think about food in new ways. And you will have to unlearn some old, outdated notions. And if you have been overweight, it is very likely that you will have to buy some new clothes!

WHAT DOES IT MEAN TO *REVERSE* DIABETES?

Most people with diabetes find themselves on a road leading towards gradually increasing weight, slowly rising blood sugar, higher doses of medications and worsening complications. Reversing diabetes means reversing this trend. If weight is an issue, it can come down – gradually, but decisively. Blood glucose values that have gone up can also come down. Doses of medications that have risen again and again can come down, too. Symptoms such as neuropathy – nerve pain in the feet and legs – can improve and even disappear. Heart disease can be reversed.

Will the disease go away completely? Some people would argue that once someone has diabetes, that person will always have it, even if blood tests improve so much that the condition is no longer diagnosable. What they mean is that the genetic traits that made type 2 diabetes possible do not go away, and type 1 diabetes requires continued insulin treatments regardless of how well you adjust your diet.

It is not possible to say in advance how far you can go. Will you be able to reduce your medication doses, eliminate some or perhaps all of your medications, or drive your blood sugar down so far that no one would ever know you once had diabetes? These are questions your own experience will answer, but I can promise this book will teach you what you need to know about putting a powerful food prescription to work. The rest of the story is yours to write.

I would be very grateful if you would let others know what you are doing and perhaps lend this book to your friends or family members who have diabetes. We know that we can turn this disease around for individuals, but conquering an international epidemic is a tall order, and it requires a team effort. I hope you will join in this important cause along with health professionals, research participants and their families.

Thank you, and the very best of luck with this programme.

PART 1

The
Breakthrough

CHAPTER 1

The Basics Have Changed

In the past few years, much of what we thought we knew about diabetes has been turned on its head. What is now coming into focus is an understanding of its fundamental *causes*, and that gives us power we never had before.

To make sure we are at the same starting point, let me talk you through the basics: symptoms, diabetes types and typical treatments as they are currently used. Then I will show you what's new.

HOW DO WE KNOW IT'S DIABETES?

First, let's make sense of the symptoms. Diabetes may arrive with no symptoms at all, but often it starts with fatigue. For no apparent reason, your spark is just no longer there. It may also seem that you are losing water more rapidly than you should be, which is to say that you make trips to the bathroom more often than usual. And you are thirsty: you find yourself drinking a surprising amount of water.

Here is what is going on: the fundamental problem is that sugar is not able to pass from your bloodstream into the cells of your body. From that single problem come a great many others, like one domino knocking over another and another and another.

The sugar we are speaking of is glucose – one of the smallest and simplest sugar molecules. In this case, *sugar* is not just another word for junk food or empty calories. The fact is that the cells of your body use this kind of sugar – glucose – as an energy source. Like petrol for your car or jet fuel for an aeroplane, glucose is your body's fuel. It powers your movements, your thoughts and more or less everything you do.

And that is exactly the problem. If glucose is unable to enter your cells, they are deprived of their basic fuel, so you lose your energy. That is why you are fatigued. If your muscles do not have the glucose they need for power, you tire easily.

Meanwhile, the glucose that cannot get into your muscle cells builds up in your bloodstream. It becomes more and more concentrated in the blood, and eventually it starts to pass through the kidneys and ends up in your urine.*

Now, as glucose passes through your kidneys, it carries water along with it – lots of water, hence all those trips to the bathroom. What follows, naturally, is thirst – you are losing all those fluids. So fatigue, frequent urination and thirst are all symptoms of one problem: glucose having trouble getting into your cells.

You may also find that you are losing weight. And no, this is not an especially welcome event – not in this situation. You lose weight because your cells are in essence starving. Nutrients cannot enter your cells, so your body is malnourished. Yes, even if you are eating plenty of food, nutrients and fuel are unable to get where they are needed.

Every day, people arrive at doctors' offices complaining of fatigue, frequent urination, thirst and sometimes unexplained weight loss. The doctor takes a blood sample, finds an unusually high level of glucose in the blood, and diagnoses diabetes. The doctor then advises the patient that it is essential to get blood sugar under control. An overly large amount of glucose flooding through the bloodstream day after day can harm the arteries. Left unchecked, it can damage the heart and the delicate blood vessels of the eyes, kidneys and extremities.

But as we have shown in our research studies, the road to high blood sugar is a two-way street. When you change your diet and make other healthy improvements, a rising glucose level can fall. Sometimes the change can be so dramatic that no doctor looking at you afterwards would ever guess that you had once been diagnosed with diabetes.

---

* The passage of glucose from the bloodstream into the urine led to the technical name doctors use for diabetes: diabetes mellitus. *Diabetes* comes from a Greek word meaning 'to pass through', and *mellitus* is the Latin word for 'honey' or 'sweet'.

How Doctors Diagnose Diabetes

Doctors diagnose diabetes if:

• You have symptoms of diabetes (frequent urination, unusual thirst, unexplained weight loss) and your blood glucose level is 11.1 millimoles per litre (mmol/l)* or higher, regardless of the time of day or whether you are fasting, or

• Your blood glucose level is 7.0 mmol/l or higher after an 8-hour fast.

Your doctor will consider this a provisional diagnosis until it is confirmed by similar testing on a separate day. In some cases, doctors perform a glucose tolerance test, in which you drink a syrup containing 75 grams of glucose. If your blood glucose value is 11.1 mmol/l or higher 2 hours later, your doctor will diagnose diabetes.

Normal fasting blood glucose is less than 5.6 mmol/l. After a 2-hour glucose tolerance test, the value should be less than 7.8 mmol/l. If your values are above the normal limit but not high enough for a diagnosis of diabetes, your doctor will diagnose prediabetes (impaired glucose tolerance), which often precedes an eventual diabetes diagnosis.

* In most countries, glucose is measured in millimoles per litre (mmol/l). In the US it is measured in milligrams per decilitre (mg/dl), therefore mg/dl is the measure you will find quoted if you look up US research or websites.

Diabetes Types

A diagnosis of diabetes – or prediabetes – means the insulin in your body is not doing its job adequately. Insulin is a hormone that moves sugar from your bloodstream into the cells of your body, among other functions. It acts like a key, opening a door to the cell, so to speak, and allowing nutrients inside. When insulin arrives at the cell's surface and opens the door, glucose is able to enter the cell, which uses it for power.

If for some reason your body is not making insulin, the result is rising blood glucose levels. Similarly, your blood glucose rises if your cells resist insulin's actions – the key goes in the lock, but the door will not open. Over the long run, high blood glucose levels can damage your nerves, eyes, kidneys and other parts of your body.

Diabetes comes in three main types, called type 1, type 2 and gestational diabetes. Let's look at each one.

Type 1 diabetes usually manifests in childhood or young adulthood. It used to be called childhood-onset or insulin-dependent diabetes. In type 1 diabetes, something has damaged the pancreas's ability to produce insulin, and you need to get it from an outside source – typically by injection. However, recent research has revealed a great deal about how diet changes can dramatically reduce the risk that diabetes will bring any serious complications your way, as you will see in Chapter 3.

In addition, we know more than ever about the causes of the disease, arming us with more power to prevent it. The damage to the insulin-producing cells is caused by the biological equivalent of 'friendly fire'. That is, it is caused by the body's immune system – our white blood cells that are supposed to fight bacteria and viruses. These cells ought to protect you, but instead they have attacked the cells of the pancreas, destroying its ability to produce insulin. In Chapter 3, we will look at what triggers this process. It may surprise you to learn that foods – particularly the foods infants are fed within the first months of life – are leading suspects.

Type 2 diabetes used to be called adult-onset diabetes, or sometimes non-insulin-dependent diabetes. About 9 out of 10 people with diabetes have type 2. Most people with this form of the disease still produce insulin; the problem is that their cells resist it. Insulin tries to bring glucose into the cells, but the cells respond like a door with a malfunctioning lock. In response to these sluggish cells, your body produces more and more insulin, trying to overcome the resistance. If the body's insulin supply cannot overcome the resistance, glucose simply builds up in your blood.

Diabetes drugs work to counteract this problem: some make your cells more responsive to insulin. Others cause your pancreas to release more insulin into the bloodstream or block your liver from sending extra glucose into the blood.

Until now, most diabetes diets have tried to compensate for the cells' resistance to insulin's action, too. They limit the amount of sugar in your diet. They also limit starch (complex carbohydrate) because starch is actually made from many glucose molecules joined together in a chain. During digestion, starch breaks down to release natural sugars into the blood. The idea is that if you do not get too much carbohydrate at any one time, your cells will not be overwhelmed with too much glucose. For people on medications, typical diet plans aim to

Insulin is Made in the Pancreas

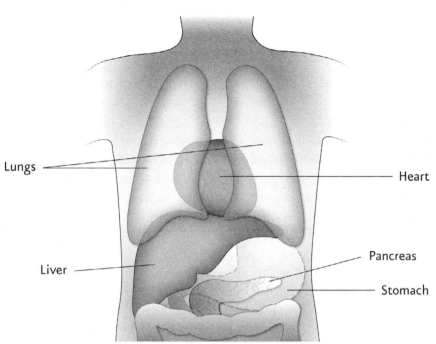

Insulin is made in the pancreas, an organ located just behind your stomach that is about the size and shape of a TV remote control. In fact, remote control is what the pancreas is all about. It sends insulin into the bloodstream to travel to the cells of your body to help them take in glucose from the bloodstream. In type 1 diabetes, the pancreas has stopped making insulin. In type 2 and gestational diabetes, the pancreas is usually able to make insulin, but the body's cells resist its action.

keep the amount of glucose or starch fairly constant from meal to meal and from day to day so the amount of medication required to help your body process glucose – your daily dosage – can stay the same, too. In short, these diets guide you on what, when and how much to eat.

New research has changed everything, however. We can now use diet changes to influence insulin sensitivity directly. So, as you will see shortly, the nutrition prescription has been completely rewritten to take advantage of this new understanding.

Gestational diabetes is similar to type 2 except that it occurs during pregnancy. While it typically disappears after childbirth, it is a sign of insulin resistance, and that means that type 2 diabetes may be around the corner. With the same sorts of steps that tackle type 2 diabetes, we can often stop gestational diabetes from ever turning into type 2.

GENES ARE NOT DESTINY

Diabetes runs in families, but don't take that to mean that if one of your parents has diabetes, a similar diagnosis has to be your fate as well. You can change things.

Let's take a look at type 1 diabetes first. Many children are born with genes that make it possible for them to develop type 1 diabetes, but most of them never do. In fact, even among identical twins, when one twin has type 1 diabetes, the other has less than a 40 per cent chance of having it.[1] What makes the difference, apparently, is the environment, particularly the foods the child is exposed to early in life, viral infections, and perhaps other factors.

Genes play a similar role in type 2 diabetes. Many years before diabetes ever manifests, special tests can detect insulin resistance in young adults who have inherited a tendency towards type 2 diabetes from their parents. If they eat the same kinds of foods their parents did, they are very likely headed for a diagnosis. Abundant evidence shows, however, that changes in diet and lifestyle can cut the odds that diabetes will occur. When it does occur, diet can dramatically alter its course.

The point is this: some genes are dictators, and others are not. The genes for hair colour or eye colour, for example, really are dictators. If they call for you to have brown hair or blue eyes, you can't argue. But the genes for diabetes are more like committees. They do not give orders; they make suggestions.

If our genes call for diabetes, we do not necessarily have to listen to them. We have more control than you might imagine.

HAEMOGLOBIN A1C

As you have seen, doctors diagnose diabetes based on your blood glucose level, and tracking your blood glucose is an important way to track the effects of diet and medication dosages. As helpful as glucose testing is, though, it really indicates only how you are doing at the time you take the test. The best way to tell how you are doing over the long run is with a test called haemoglobin A1c, or HbA1c. This is the main way you will track your progress in controlling diabetes.

Haemoglobin is the pigment that gives colour to your red blood cells and whose job it is to carry oxygen. What the HbA1c test actually measures is how much glucose has entered your red blood cells and become stuck to haemoglobin. If you have had a lot of glucose in your blood, a fair amount of it gets into your cells and sticks to your haemoglobin. If you have not had much glucose in your blood, your haemoglobin has much less stuck to it.

Since red blood cells have a fairly short life span (about 4 months), the test indicates how well your blood sugar has been controlled over the preceding 3 months or so. According to Diabetes UK, people with diabetes should aim for an HbA1c of 6.5 per cent or below, as research shows that this lowers the risk of complications.

DIABETES DIETS

If you have diabetes, chances are you were given printed guidelines on what to eat and what to avoid. Perhaps you have met with a dietitian, and you may have been referred to a diabetes class. Unfortunately, most people do not get the ongoing support they need to make dietary changes, and as a result, this well-meaning effort may not have much effect. If you are like many people, you may have found your diet tough to sustain.

For many years, Diabetes UK – in line with similar authorities in most Western countries – has recommended eating habits designed to provide basic nutrition while also keeping calorie intake and food choices reasonably stable over the course of the day and from one day to the next, as you saw above. The idea was that if you had no carbohydrates for breakfast but then had a big carb-fest later in the day, your blood sugar would change erratically. Similarly, if you had lots of starchy foods on Monday but went low-carb the rest of the week, your blood sugar would be all over the map, and your medications could not keep up with you.

In the UK, your general practitioner will ask you to meet the practice nurse specialist in diabetes, who will, either herself or with a dietitian, provide an individualized plan describing specific numbers of servings of various foods for your meals and snacks, taking into account both your need to reduce your weight or cholesterol and your use of medications. In other countries, dietary plans are provided by specialist diabetes centres. Within your plan, you would be able to choose foods using 'exchange lists'. That is, if the dietitian prescribed a certain number of starch servings at breakfast, for example, you could decide whether that starch is one-quarter of a roll, one slice of raisin bread, ½ cup of cereal or any other choice on the starch exchange list. Likewise, if your meal plan called for you to have a piece of fruit, you could pick from a range of choices with similar nutritional makeups.

Following this advice does improve most people's eating habits. (If you would like to put yourself in the hands of a registered dietitian with special interest in diabetes your doctor can arrange an appointment.) The results of this approach vary dramatically from one person to the next, however. Some lose weight and see their glucose numbers fall; others don't get too far. In research studies, the typical drop in HbA1c – the indicator of blood sugar control discussed above – is roughly 0.5 percentage point (e.g., from 8.0 to 7.5 per cent), with some studies showing slightly better results and others worse (you will learn more about HbA1c and other tests in Chapter 7).[2-4]

Researchers and doctors have long lamented these lacklustre results. In 1993, an article in the *Journal of the American Dietetic Association* summed up the findings of research studies up to that point and concluded that diabetes diets are challenging and most people do not follow them.[5] Experience of doctors in many countries is similar. The guidelines are understandable and, to an extent, logical, but even with a fair amount of support, many people find it hard to make the diet work in their day-to-day lives.

The diet you will read about in this book is completely different. For many people, it is much easier as well as much more effective and up-to-date. Now, consulting a registered dietitian is still a good idea because he or she can guide you in the approach described in the following chapters. Take this book with you; your dietitian can help you get started.

DRUGS AND MONEY

The diet you will read about in this book is powerful. Unfortunately, the power of nutrition is neglected in many medical practices, and in the process, diabetes treatment is reduced to a series of prescriptions.

Don't misunderstand me. Diabetes medications can be lifesaving. They can reduce your blood sugar and, over the long run, cut your risk of complications. And if diet and lifestyle changes do not do the job, it is a serious mistake to forgo medications (you can find a detailed description of them in Appendix 1). But some doctors and patients view medications as the only tools at their disposal. The marketing of pharmaceuticals has been so successful that many doctors give little more than lip service to diet and exercise, which can often be dramatically effective.

Open any diabetes journal and you will see expensive advertisements for this drug and that drug.

If you were to leaf through the post that floods doctors' surgeries, you would see information about medical courses, symposia and online educational programmes, all paid for by drug companies trumpeting their products. These companies make great efforts to lure doctors to presentations about one or another application of their drugs. While many US doctors find this distasteful, in many cases they are required to attend medical courses to maintain their hospital or university affiliations, and drug companies have cornered the medical education market. In the UK the situation is a little different. In the past, pressure from pharmaceutical companies has perhaps led to doctors putting more emphasis on drugs, rather than diet and lifestyle, as the main approach to diabetes treatment. Today, however, the organizers of continuing training for British doctors understand the need to differentiate between sponsorship of meetings and the promotion of drugs, with the result that medical meetings in the UK are less influenced by commercial interests.

It is my hope that as the power of nutritional changes is more fully appreciated, doctors will begin to focus on diet even more, educating parents about nutritional approaches to help prevent type 1 diabetes in their children, and working with schools to serve healthy meals so children are not sent down the road to overweight and diabetes, as a great many currently are. These measures could control the so-called diseases of affluence far more effectively than doctors are able to at present, dramatically reducing the need for medications in the first place.

Each person with diabetes has a unique ability to heal and return to health. This ability differs from one person to the next, but in our studies, we have not seen age, weight or any other factor to be a barrier to improvement.

The remainder of this book will show you what I believe to be the most powerful dietary approach to diabetes that is currently known.

CHAPTER 2

Reversing Type 2 Diabetes

Remarkably, my research has shown that it is possible to reverse diabetes – to decrease blood sugar, medication doses and the risk of complications – and this chapter will show you how, using surprisingly simple diet changes. I will also share some surprising new findings about the causes of type 2 diabetes – changes inside your body's cells that can be detected years before diabetes starts. Evidence suggests that switching to a healthier diet has a powerful influence on the workings of your cells, as you will see.

All doctors and dietitians recognize that if you have diabetes, your body does not process sugar very well, which is to say that the amount of sugar in your bloodstream is too high. Researchers learned long ago that if it stays high, you are at risk of many health problems down the road.

To lower your blood sugar, most medical professionals are likely to prescribe a diet that includes very little sugar. They will also ask you to limit starchy foods – such as bread, potatoes, rice and pasta – because in your digestive tract, starch breaks apart to release sugar (that is, glucose). It seems to make sense – if your body cannot handle sugar, you have to be careful about eating too much sugar and anything that turns into it. Your medical team will also encourage you to space out your intake of starches and sugars throughout the day – and from one day to the next – so that it stays fairly even over time. Diabetes diets also generally cut calories to help you lose weight and limit certain fats to reduce the risk of heart disease and other complications. That, in a nutshell, is a typical 'traditional' diabetes diet.

It is certainly logical, and some people greatly benefit from following it. The problem is that for most people, this sort of diet change has only a very limited effect. Weight loss is usually modest, and the diet alone typically is not enough to bring blood sugar under control.

Sooner or later, you and your doctor are likely to decide that the 'diabetes diet' is not helping very much, and your doctor will add various drugs. You may need one, two or even three different oral medications. Eventually, your doctor may consider adding insulin injections. And because many people with diabetes also have high blood pressure or high cholesterol levels, doctors often add medications to tackle these problems, too. Instead of helping you reduce or avoid medications, the diet seems to be a stepping-stone on the way to an ever-increasing list of drugs.

The first glimmer that there might be a better way came from a look at the prevalence of diabetes around the world. Large population studies showed that diabetes was rare in Japan, China, Thailand and other Asian countries. It was similarly rare in parts of Africa.

These studies also showed something else: people in countries where diabetes was uncommon were not following anything like a 'diabetes diet'. They did not avoid carbohydrates; they ate starchy foods every day. In Asia and Africa, rice and other grains, starchy vegetables, bean dishes and noodles are staples. In fact, researchers found that people in these countries ate considerably more carbohydrates than Europeans or North Americans do, yet diabetes was relatively rare. So were weight problems. While obesity is found in more than 20 per cent of British adults and 30 per cent of American adults, it occurred in less than 1 per cent of Japanese adults following a traditional diet. Heart disease and several forms of cancer were rare, too. Longevity among Japanese adults was better than that of Europeans or North Americans.

That is, until they moved to the US. For a Japanese adult, a move to North America dramatically increased the risk of diabetes. Heart disease, obesity and other problems became much more common, too.

Now, if you are worrying that I am going to ask you to adopt a traditional Japanese diet, relax. That's not a bad idea, but it is not what this book is about. I raise this international comparison simply to make an important point: *carbohydrates do not cause diabetes*. And a diet that focuses on keeping carbohydrates out of your diet is not a powerful way to manage – let alone reverse – the disease. If anything, healthy complex carbohydrates help prevent it.

Think about what happens when an Asian man or woman switches to a Western lifestyle. Hamburgers, fried chicken, cheese and other Western fare come into the diet, while rice and noodles are gradually forgotten. The diet becomes fattier and much higher in protein, while carbohydrate-rich rice and noodles and other starchy foods fall by the wayside.

Tragically, that is exactly what is happening. What's more, Asian men and women need not leave home for these changes to occur. McDonald's has come to them; Burger King, KFC and other Western eating habits have also invaded Asia. Meat, cheese and other greasy foods are displacing rice and vegetables.

As the Japanese diet has become Westernized, the prevalence of diabetes has exploded. In studies of adults in Japan over the age of 40, diabetes prevalence was between 1 and 5 per cent prior to 1980. By 1990, it had gone up to 11 to 12 per cent.[1] Statistical projections suggest it will rise even further. It turns out that the genes that allow diabetes to occur are surprisingly common among the Japanese, but as long as they stuck to their rice-based traditional diet, the disease was mostly held in check. The diabetes genes lay dormant, like seeds on dry soil. Once rice fell out of fashion and Western eating habits took hold, the genetic traits started to show themselves.

So, if people in Asia or Africa who eat lots of carbohydrates have very little diabetes, and if the disease becomes more and more common as carbohydrates are excluded from the diet, researchers have had to conclude that a high-carbohydrate diet is not the cause of the disease. In fact, the culprit seems to be lurking in our Western diets.

The inescapable fact is that the problem is not carbohydrates (that is, sugar and starch). *The problem is in how the body processes them.* If we can repair your body's ability to absorb and use carbohydrates, not only can you enjoy healthy carbohydrate-rich foods without worry, but diabetes itself ought to improve – perhaps even go away.

A look inside your body will show you what I mean.

A LOOK INSIDE YOUR BODY

Your pancreas, an organ in your abdomen, produces insulin. As you know by now, insulin is a hormone, and the pancreas sends it into your bloodstream to travel to the various cells of the body. Like a key sliding into a lock, insulin attaches to a receptor on the cell's surface and causes the cell membrane to permit glucose to enter. Insulin does the same thing for the next cell, and the next, and the next. It attaches to a receptor on the cell's surface, opens the door and ushers glucose in.

In type 2 diabetes, this system does not work properly. Your pancreas makes insulin, and insulin travels to each cell, but when it arrives, it has trouble opening the door. It is as if the lock has somehow become jammed and the key no longer works. This is insulin resistance. Yes, the insulin 'key' is there, but it has trouble doing its job. Glucose cannot get into the cells and it builds up in the bloodstream.

Imagine the workings of a lock on a typical door. What if someone were to jam chewing gum into the lock? There is nothing wrong with your key and really nothing wrong with the lock except that it is now filled with gum. To make it work again, we need to clean it out.

The new approach to diabetes is based on cleaning out your biological locks. Our goal is to help your insulin 'key' work the way it is supposed to.

THE NEW DIABETES DIET

As far back as the early 1900s, researchers were adjusting people's diets to try to improve insulin sensitivity.[2,3] Over the years, many – like me – have been inspired by the fact that foods that are commonly eaten in Asia or Africa somehow help prevent diabetes.

In 1979, researchers at the University of Kentucky studied 20 men with type 2 diabetes, all of whom had been taking an average of 26 units of insulin per day. The experimental diet included plenty of vegetables, fruits, whole grains and beans, so it was high in fibre and carbohydrate. The diet was nearly vegetarian, with very little animal fat – in fact, very little fat of any kind.

After just 16 days on the programme, more than half of the men were able to stop taking insulin entirely, and their blood sugar levels were *lower* than before.[4] For the remaining men, insulin doses were cut dramatically. That was an amazing and rapid result. But the study was short, and the participants lived on the research ward for its duration. It was unclear whether a similar result would be seen in people living on their own and preparing their own meals and whether it would be sustained over the long term.

A study conducted at the University of California, Los Angeles – 197 men enrolled in a 3-week diet change and exercise programme – showed much the same thing. Of this group, 140 were able to discontinue their medications.[5] That was a great result and it occurred very quickly. The study's limitation from our point of view was that it could not separate the effects of diet from those of exercise. Both are important, of course, but if we want to track down the best diet for diabetes, it is important to keep everything else constant while the diet is being tested.

Several years ago, my research team began a series of studies to see what diet alone could do. We tested a diet that focused not on limiting carbohydrates but rather on getting as much fat off the plate as possible. We thought if we could do that, perhaps we could clean out the 'lock' mechanism that opens the cell doors.

We began with a small pilot study, which I mentioned briefly in the introduction. Most of the participants were surprised to see rice, pasta, sweet potatoes and beans on the menu and even more surprised that the diet did not limit carbohydrates at all. No matter how long they had had diabetes or how nervous they felt about the idea of putting carbohydrates back on to their plates, we put no limit on carbs at all.

There was also no limit on portions. Most of our participants were overweight, but we did not ask them to limit portions or cut calories.

What we zeroed in on was fat. We aimed to clean all the grease out of the participants' diets. So, instead of bacon and eggs for breakfast, they had to choose from old-fashioned oats, half a cantaloupe or wholemeal toast. If they had chilli for lunch, it was veggie chilli. Instead of pasta topped with meat sauce, they got meatless marinara. For the duration of the study, we asked them to set aside animal products completely and stick to vegetarian foods.

Needless to say, if there are no animal products in the diet, there is not a single drop of animal fat. We kept the use of vegetable oils as minimal as possible, too. And, in order to isolate the effects of the diet, we asked the participants not to alter their normal activity patterns; no one was to add exercise to the regime. Now, exercise is an important part of any healthy lifestyle, and ordinarily we would strongly encourage it. But this was a test of the diet alone, and for scientific reasons, exercise was not to be part of it.

At the end of the study period, everyone weighed in. In just 12 weeks, the average participant had lost 7.2 kg (1 st 2 lb). Their fasting blood sugar had dropped 28 per cent. Two-thirds of the participants on diabetes medications were able to reduce or discontinue them in that short period of time.[6] All this occurred without any limits on calories, portions or carbohydrates and without exercise. These effects were significantly greater than those seen in a control group carefully following the diet guidelines of the American Diabetes Association (ADA).

That was impressive. But *why* did it happen? How does a diet that gives a green light to pasta, rice and all the other foods that people with diabetes thought they had to live without – and one that completely disregards calories and avoids exercise – cause blood sugar to plummet and weight to easily drop away?

To answer that question, we designed another study. This one included a group of women who were moderately or severely overweight but did not have diabetes. Once again, we zeroed in on animal fat and vegetable oils. Our participants set animal products aside and kept oils to a bare minimum. And they were free to implement the diet guidelines in their own way, whether they ate at home or ate out, so it was a good test of how the diet would work in real life. For one person, eating out might have meant mushroom stroganoff with steamed vegetables; for another, it might have been vegetable sushi with miso soup and salad. As long as they avoided animal products and kept oils to a minimum, they were free to shape their meals to their liking.

For comparison, we included a control group whose members followed what you might think of as a typical cholesterol-lowering diet. It cut back on red meat while emphasizing poultry and fish along with plenty of vegetables, fruits and whole grains.

The results were quick and impressive. The vegetarian group participants lost about 0.5 kg (1 lb) per week; after 14 weeks, they had lost an average of nearly 6 kg (13 lb), compared to almost half that for the control group.[7]

By now, it was no surprise that this diet causes weight loss, but we went a step further. We sent our participants to the laboratory for a glucose tolerance test, which allowed us to measure how their bodies responded to sugar and how well their bodies' insulin was working. Each participant swallowed a dose of sugary syrup, and we took blood samples every half hour to measure rises in blood sugar and insulin. From these laboratory data, we were able to calculate each woman's insulin sensitivity and track how it changed as the study progressed.

The results were remarkable. The tests showed that our participants were physically changing. Based on their laboratory measurements, it was clear that their bodies' cells were becoming more and more sensitive to insulin. By the 14-week point, their insulin sensitivity had improved by 24 per cent. In other words, something about the diet reactivated their natural insulin's ability to open cell doors to glucose. What that means, of course, is that the diet was addressing the fundamental problem we see in type 2 diabetes: it was helping glucose get to where it belonged.*

Based on these and other studies, the National Institutes of Health – the research branch of the US government – decided to fund a new study. Working with me on the project were researchers from George Washington University School of Medicine and the University of Toronto and dietitians and physicians working with the Physicians Committee for Responsible Medicine, a nonprofit organization I founded in 1985.

The study included 99 people with type 2 diabetes. For 22 weeks, 49 of them followed a diet that was similar to those we had tested earlier. The diet was vegan – meaning that it included no animal products at all – and was low in fat. Also, while we placed no limits on the amount

---

* The study turned up another particularly remarkable finding. In a laboratory at George Washington University, we measured the participants' metabolism – how fast their bodies burned calories. This was done by measuring how much oxygen they consumed minute by minute and how much carbon dioxide they produced after being given a test meal (two cans of a standard liquid formula).

After 14 weeks on the experimental diet, it was clear that the participants had a significant increase in their after-meal calorie burn; their after-meal calorie-burning speed increased by 16 per cent.[8]

What was happening was that the diet had made their cells more sensitive to insulin's action, so they were able to take in nutrients more quickly. Glucose got out of the blood and into the cells, where more of it could be burned up, so to speak. These calories are released as body heat rather than being stored as body fat. Scientists call this the thermic effect of food, and it provides a small extra edge for weight loss.

of carbohydrates our participants could have, we encouraged everyone to be selective about the kinds of carbohydrates they ate. Instead of white bread, we encouraged them to choose rye or pumpernickel. Instead of baking potatoes, we favoured sweet potatoes. The remaining 50 participants followed a diet based on the ADA guidelines. Once again, we restricted exercise.

Over the ensuing weeks, many participants found their blood sugar falling to the extent that they had to cut back on their diabetes medications. That was a happy outcome, but it was not our goal. In fact, we were trying to keep medications unchanged as much as we could so we could isolate the effect of the diet on their blood sugar. The combination of the diet and the blood sugar–lowering drugs was so powerful, however, that many participants *had* to reduce their doses or discontinue medications altogether to keep their blood sugar from dropping too low.

To really gauge what the diet could do, we looked at those participants whose medications had stayed constant and how the diet affected HbA1c – the principal gauge of blood glucose control. The ADA diet had reduced HbA1c by 0.4 percentage point – a good change. But the vegan diet was three times more effective. It had reduced HbA1c by 1.2 percentage points (the average person's value fell from 8.0 to 6.8 per cent during the 22-week study). That is a stronger effect than is seen with a typical diabetes medication. The common diabetes drug metformin (Glucophage), for example, reduced HbA1c by about 0.6 percentage point in a large research trial.[9] The vegan diet also proved highly effective in reducing body weight and cholesterol.

To put all this in perspective, the landmark UK Prospective Diabetes Study showed that a 1-point drop in HbA1c for people with type 2 diabetes lowers the risk of eye or kidney complications by about 37 per cent.[10] This is the effect of just the HbA1c drop without considering the ability of the diet to also reduce cholesterol and blood pressure.[11]

In the next chapter, I will show you how you can test this diet to see what it can do for you. But let's look a bit closer at the science behind this approach.

TOWARDS THE PERFECT DIET

Setting aside animal products and keeping oily foods to a minimum may sound challenging, but our participants commonly reported just the opposite. One man, Walter, said, 'I'm amazed at how easy it was to adapt to this diet. And I feel great. Within 2 months, I lost 20 pounds [9 kg]. And the more amazing thing to me is that my glucose averages have fallen by 30 to 40 [1.7 to 2.2] points.'

For Mark, the change was 'an adventure. I tried new restaurants, new recipes and different foods I would never have eaten before. My main goal was to lose weight, and I've lost a good 30 pounds [13.6 kg] so far. When I started, my fasting blood sugar was 260 to 360 [14.4 to 20]. And it dropped like a rock. Now I'm between 130 and 135 [7.2 and 7.5]. And I don't get tired in the afternoon like I used to.'

Nancy agreed. She felt totally adjusted to the diet within about 30 days. 'And within 5 months of making the change,' she said, 'my blood sugar fell so much that I was able to stop one of my medications. I have much more energy and really feel tremendous.'

I will take you through the diet step by step. If it sounds like a very healthy diet, it certainly is – and not just for controlling blood sugar.

In 1990, Dr Dean Ornish, a young Harvard-trained physician, discovered a remarkable feature of a low-fat, vegetarian diet. He tested the diet in individuals with heart disease and added other healthy lifestyle changes – regular exercise, stress modification and smoking cessation. Because the diet contained no animal products, it had no cholesterol at all and very little fat. After a year's time, each patient had a special x-ray of the heart called an angiogram, and Dr Ornish's team compared the results with angiograms done on the same patients at the beginning of the study. The results made medical history. The patients' coronary arteries, which had been blocked by years of poor diet, were actually starting to open again. The difference was clearly visible in 82 per cent of the patients after 1 year. This occurred without surgery or drugs – even without cholesterol-lowering medication.[12,13]

Other researchers have shown that this same sort of diet change reduces blood pressure. Apparently, eliminating animal fats reduces the viscosity ('thickness') of the blood. That is, the blood becomes less like grease and more like water, so it easily flows through the arteries, causing blood pressure to fall. Blood pressure is also reduced by the potassium in vegetables and fruits, and other characteristics of plant foods augment this benefit.[14]

Vegetarians are slimmer, too. The average person who embraces a vegetarian diet loses about 10 per cent of his or her body weight.

These changes would be welcomed by most of us, but if you have diabetes, they can be lifesaving. This is because, as you saw in Chapter 1, persistently high blood sugar can attack the blood vessels of your heart, eyes, kidneys and legs. What kills most people who have diabetes (that is, those who have not made the diet changes you are reading about) is damage to their hearts. A diet that reverses that process – turning the clock backwards on heart disease, reducing blood pressure and trimming weight – is powerful medicine for everyone with diabetes, whether type 1 or type 2.

Imagine if your eyes were damaged by the disease. An ophthalmologic surgeon, laser in hand, would carefully try to repair your tender retinas. But what if foods could help avert this damage in the first place? A diet change that brings your blood sugar under control, brings your blood pressure down, and helps rejuvenate your arteries gives a measure of respite to the tiny blood vessels in your eyes. It does the same for the tiny vessels that make up the filtering unit in your kidneys, making it less likely that you will ever need dialysis. And of course, it works powerfully inside the heart.

Now, do not misunderstand me. I am not suggesting that you should forgo needed medical treatments and rely on diet alone. But a diet change – if it goes far enough and begins early enough – can revolutionize your health, dramatically cut your risk of complications and even reverse these complications to a degree.

INSIDE THE CELL

In discussing type 2 diabetes, I have described each cell of the body as being rather like a gummed-up lock. Research has shown this analogy to be surprisingly apt. Indeed, insulin's ability to work is blocked by the accumulation of something within the cells: not gum, but fat.

In the February 12, 2004, issue of the *New England Journal of Medicine,* Yale University researchers reported an amazing discovery.[15] They tested young adults whose parents or grandparents had had type 2 diabetes. All were thin and healthy, and none had diabetes at that point. But some were insulin resistant, meaning that when they were given a test dose of glucose, it built up more than it should have in their bloodstream. The researchers found out why: inside their muscle cells were tiny amounts of fat, fat that interfered with insulin's ability to work.

Their bodies made insulin normally, and it reached their muscle cells with no problem. Once it got there, though, it did not work properly. The muscle cells simply could not fully respond to insulin because they contained bits of fat, like gum jammed in a lock rendering a key useless.

How did this fat get there? Well, muscle cells normally store a tiny amount of fat, which provides an energy source for physical activity. The amount is normally quite small, and the fat simply waits for that day when you are much more active than usual and need a bit of extra energy. For some reason, in these young people, fat had built up much more than it should have – to levels 80 per cent higher than in other young people. The fat buildup had reached the point where it was gumming up the lock. That is, it was interfering with the cell's ability to respond to insulin, and that meant that diabetes was very likely in their future unless something changed in a major way.

Fat Inside Cells Interferes with Insulin's Action

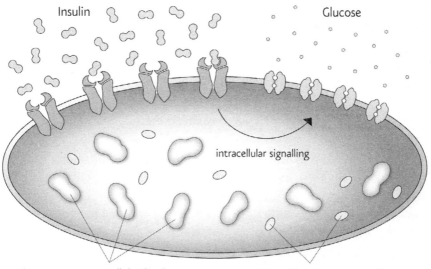

Normally, insulin attaches to receptors on the cell's surface and signals the cell membrane to allow glucose to enter. However, if fat, called intramyocellular lipid, accumulates inside the cell, it interferes with insulin's intracellular signalling process. Tiny organelles, called mitochondria, are supposed to burn fat, and their failure to keep up with the accumulating fat may be the origin of type 2 diabetes. Luckily, evidence shows that diet changes can reduce the amount of fat inside the cell.

I should emphasize that the fat inside your cells is different from the fat around your waistline. Even if you are quite slim, you may still be accumulating fat within your muscle cells. The participants in the Yale study *were* slim, averaging only 64 kg (10 st). They were young and healthy. But just as young people who smoke are setting the stage for cancer decades later, young people who accumulate fat inside their muscle cells are paving the way for diabetes.

Until now, diabetes diets have not been designed to alter what goes on inside the cells. Instead, they have been designed to compensate for the problem, so to speak. Because your cells cannot handle glucose – that is, insulin has trouble getting glucose into them – the diets limit sugars and foods that contain carbohydrate, because when carbohydrate is digested, it releases sugars. But what if a change in diet could actually alter the fat buildup within the cells and reverse the trend towards gradually worsening insulin resistance?

I believe this is exactly what we can do – exactly what you *will* do as you make the diet changes described in this book. But first, a few more details from inside the cells.

TINY FURNACES THAT BURN FAT

There is a term for the tiny bits of fat that build up inside muscle cells. Scientists call them intramyocellular lipids (*intra-* means 'inside', *myo-* is 'muscle' and *lipid* is 'fat' – literally, fat inside muscle cells). As you have seen, these traces of fat start accumulating many years before diabetes manifests.[16]

Let's go one step further and look at how the fat builds up. Your cells have microscopic 'furnaces' or 'burners' that are supposed to metabolize bits of fat and convert it into energy. If all is operating normally, fat enters the cell and these tiny burners use it up. These burners are called mitochondria, and they are responsible for turning fat or other fuel sources into energy to power your muscle cells. If you are steadily accumulating fat, that is a sign that your burners – your mitochondria – are falling down on the job.

In type 2 diabetes, the problem appears to be too few mitochondria. That is, people with type 2 diabetes have fewer mitochondria than they need to burn up the accumulating fat. If they had more of these little 'furnaces' inside each cell, things would be very different.

Surprisingly enough, it may be that the number of mitochondria you have depends on what you eat. Let me describe a second research study.

At Pennington Biomedical Research Center in Baton Rouge, Louisiana, researchers studied 10 young men. They averaged just 23 years of age; were reasonably trim, averaging 78.3 kg (12 st 4 lb); and were healthy. The researchers put them on a high-fat diet that drew about half its calories from fats.[17] This is much more fat than you would want to have in your diet, but it is not far different from what many people actually eat. After just 3 days on a high-fat diet, the men had accumulated significantly more intramyocellular lipids, so the first lesson of this study was that fat builds up quickly. Depending on the foods you eat, you can pack fat into your cells surprisingly rapidly.

Then the researchers tested the genes that produce mitochondria. Just as you have genes in your cells that allow you to make bones, hormones, skin, hair and all the other structures of your body, you also have genes that serve as blueprints for mitochondria. It turned out that the fatty foods these volunteers ate did more than just pack fat into their cells; they actually *turned off the genes that would help burn fat*. The genes that produce mitochondria were in fact partially disabled. It was as if the men's bodies were trying to avoid burning the fat they had eaten so they could save it inside the cells for future use.

Imagine what this means: you have eaten fatty foods and, as a result, tiny bits of fat have accumulated in your muscle cells. This fat interferes with the normal workings of the cells, including their ability to respond to insulin. If insulin is unable to work, glucose cannot get into the cells and it builds up in the bloodstream. Then, those fatty foods actually seem to disable your genes that would produce the mitochondria you need to burn up this accumulating fat. Your ability to eliminate fat inside your cells seems to be slowed down when you eat fatty foods.

Let me speculate about why all this occurs.

Your body chemistry began to take shape many thousands of years ago, long before fast-food restaurants and convenience stores ever got their first deliveries of cheese and oil. Our human ancestors did not find fatty foods growing on trees – or at least not many of them. On the rare occasions when they ate fatty foods – meat, eggs, nuts or avocados, for example – their bodies may actually have tried to save some of the fat from these foods in case they needed it to power their muscles or food became scarce. Thus, it would not be surprising if a sudden influx of fat in the muscle cells signals them to *turn off* the fat-burning mitochondria and save the fat for future needs. Today, of course, that is the last thing we want. We want to power up our mitochondria – turn on those little furnaces to eliminate fat.

Well, can you get rid of this fat? Let's say you stopped eating fatty foods. Would intramyocellular lipid start to disappear?

Let me share the results of a startling experiment. At Catholic University in Rome, Italy, eight patients underwent gastric bypass surgery.[18] The operation is commonly done as a last-ditch treatment for massive obesity, and for good reason. What it involves is this: the stomach is stapled so that only a tiny pouch about the size of an egg is left to receive food. Then the intestine is cut in two. The first part of the intestine simply lies unused, while the lower portion of the small intestine is attached directly to the tiny stomach pouch. In this way, the patient cannot eat much food, and there is much less intestine available to absorb the nutrients from whatever food is eaten.

After the procedure, the patients were essentially starving. They could eat very little food at any given meal and any fats they ate were poorly absorbed because the first part of the small intestine, which is where fats are absorbed, was no longer connected to the stomach.

As you might imagine, they lost weight, dropping from an average of more than 137 kg (21 st) to 104 kg (16 st 4 lb) in the first 6 months. That is not unusual after such drastic surgery. What was striking was the effect on their cells. The fat inside their muscle cells – their intramyocellular lipid – dropped by 87 per cent. And even though they were still overweight, their insulin resistance had largely disappeared.

I am not recommending that you have this procedure. I am presenting these findings to make a critically important point: the fat inside your cells is not a permanent fixture. If the influx of fat stops, the fat inside the cells dissipates, and when that happens, *the cells start to regain their normal function.*

Surgery is a drastic solution, but the Italian researchers also tested whether a low-calorie diet without surgery could deplete intramyocellular lipid – and it did. Following a 1,200-calorie diet for 6 months, the patients lost about 13.6 kg (2 st) on average and eliminated about 8 per cent of the fat inside their cells. Now, that modest result came from a diet that focused just on cutting calories rather than on eating particular *types* of food, which will be the focus of this programme. The next step is to make the diet more powerful so it works a little more like surgery, without all the obvious risks of an operation.

Let's go a step further. At Imperial College School of Medicine in London, researchers studied a group of individuals following a vegan diet. They compared the participants to others who were similar in age and body weight but were not following a vegan diet.[19] When the researchers measured the intramyocellular lipid in each participant's calf muscles, they found it was 31 per cent lower in the vegans than in the omnivores. It looks as if there is something about the diet that helps prevent fat buildup in cells.

These studies show – loudly and clearly – that the accumulation of fat in the cells and all the problems it causes are not simply a matter of genes. Genes do play a role, but these effects are very much a matter of diet, too, and *it can change dramatically*.

In Part 2, you will see how to select foods to address this problem in the most powerful way possible.

CHAPTER 3

A Revolution in Type 1 Diabetes

If you have type 1 diabetes, the diet changes you will soon learn about can be lifesaving. No doubt you have heard that type 1 diabetes increases the risk of heart problems and other complications. When you really take control, however, all these risks plummet.

Research has proven that *you are not powerless to resist the complications of diabetes*. There is a lot you can do to protect yourself.

The Diabetes Control and Complications Trial did it with medication. The study was sponsored by the US government and included 1,441 people with type 1 diabetes. Some of the participants took insulin once or twice daily, as is common practice. The remaining participants were asked to follow a more intensive programme. They took insulin three or four times daily, either by injection or via an insulin pump. They checked their blood glucose several times a day and adjusted their insulin doses accordingly. Over 17 years of follow-up, the extra care these individuals took paid off dramatically. Careful tracking of blood sugar and medication adjustments lowered the risk of heart problems by 50 per cent.[1]

Also, although people with diabetes are at risk of eye problems, careful blood glucose control reduced that risk by 76 per cent compared to people on traditional medical therapy. It cut the risk of kidney problems by 39 per cent and reduced the risk of neuropathy by 60 per cent.[2]

The study treatment involved medication rather than diet, but it proved a vitally important point. Many people had imagined that diabetes complications are simply inevitable; this study showed otherwise.

Gaining control over your blood glucose makes an enormous difference. Now, with type 1 diabetes, you will need to use insulin to achieve that goal. But diet and exercise offer additional ways that too few people take advantage of. And diet is the focus of this book.

Also, it is important to understand that blood sugar control – as vital as it is – is just one part of the equation. Your risk of developing problems with your heart, kidneys, eyes or extremities also depends on your blood pressure, cholesterol levels and other factors. The goal now is to adjust your diet to control all of these to the extent that we can, adding medications as necessary according to your doctor's advice.

TOWARDS AN OPTIMAL DIET

In type 1 diabetes, your greatest risk is to your heart and blood vessels. If you do nothing, cardiovascular disease lies in wait. In fact, it strikes the majority of people with type 1 diabetes. We now have a better understanding than ever before about how to use diet and lifestyle changes to protect the heart, not only for people with diabetes but for anyone. Chapters 4 and 5 will cover how and what to eat in great detail, and Chapters 12 and 13 will discuss the complications head on. In the meantime, here are the keys.

A healthy diet. Follow the diet steps outlined in the next chapter. These practices eliminate cholesterol and animal fat, keep fats in general very low, and guide you away from sugar and refined carbohydrates and towards healthy complex carbohydrates.

As you will see, there is a special advantage to a vegetarian diet, or I should say a *vegan* diet – meaning a menu that includes no animal products at all. Dietary cholesterol is found only in animal products.*

Animal foods also tend to be high in the saturated ('bad') fats that tend to cause your body to make additional cholesterol. A vegetarian diet eliminates these problems. It has another major benefit as well: it derives all its protein from plants rather than from animal products.

---

* It is a good idea to eliminate cholesterol from your diet completely. There is no 'good' cholesterol in foods. Rather, cholesterol in foods always tends to increase your blood cholesterol level. This is in contrast to cholesterol that is measured by blood tests, which doctors separate into 'good' (HDL) and 'bad' (LDL) cholesterol, among other forms. HDL cholesterol is 'good' because it is leaving the body.

Research studies have shown that among people with any degree of kidney damage, animal protein increases the risk of further kidney deterioration.[3] On the other hand, healthy beans, grains and vegetables are just what your kidneys ordered.

Please read the next chapters very carefully. They will show you how to begin.

No smoking. If you smoke, now is the time to stop. If you have tried 50 times, it is time for try number 51. You can and will succeed. Ask your doctor to help you.

Regular exercise. Even modest exercise, such as daily walking, makes a big difference. See your doctor, who will assess your heart, your joints and your overall health to make sure you are ready for exercise. See Chapter 11 for ways to get started.

Stress management. Stress affects your health directly, causing fight-or-flight hormones to flood into your bloodstream. In turn, these hormones typically raise your blood sugar. Stress also disrupts your eating routines and interferes with sleep.

Getting a handle on stress does not mean stepping back from the challenges of life. It means finding ways to enjoy life fully without letting stress get out of control. There are many healthy ways to relax, including meditation, yoga and even simple breathing exercises.

As you saw in the previous chapter, Dr Dean Ornish showed that these four steps – a healthy vegetarian diet, smoking cessation, regular exercise and stress management – can actually reverse heart disease, even without the use of cholesterol-lowering medications. That is a tremendous benefit. Your doctor may add medications to your regime to protect you further.

These lifestyle changes will not eliminate the need to use insulin for type 1 diabetes. But they can help you stay healthy, minimizing the effects of diabetes on your life.

A NEW UNDERSTANDING OF THE CAUSES OF TYPE 1 DIABETES

Let's think for a moment beyond improving the health of people with type 1 diabetes. What if we could actually prevent it in the first place? Research over the past 2 decades suggests that we may already have the ability to prevent many cases of type 1 diabetes.

If you thought the disease was simply genetic and there was no way to stop it, read on. Studies of identical twins have set that notion aside. Identical twins, of course, have exactly the same genes, so they have the same hair colour, eye colour and facial features. If a disease were simply genetic, then, both twins would have it. But type 1 diabetes does not work that way. As I mentioned in Chapter 1, if one twin has diabetes, the other has less than a 40 per cent chance of developing it.

Thus, although genes play a role, it is clear that type 1 diabetes is not simply a genetic disease. Something else triggers it – something in the child's early environment.

For many years, researchers have known that type 1 diabetes occurs when the immune system attacks and destroys the insulin-producing cells in the pancreas. Your immune system, of course, is your defence against viruses, bacteria and cancer cells. It is not supposed to attack your own healthy body tissues, but that is exactly what occurs in type 1 diabetes.

To understand why this happens, let's look at a few basics. The complex defence network of your immune system is made up of specialized white blood cells. Some of these cells engulf invading germs and digest them. Others make antibodies – molecules that attach to invading organisms like harpoons and identify them for other immune cells to attack. If you have type 1 diabetes, your immune system has made a major error: it has attacked and destroyed your insulin-producing cells, making it what scientists call an autoimmune disease.

But why does it occur? Back in 1992, a team of Canadian and Finnish researchers reported an important discovery in the *New England Journal of Medicine*. Examining blood samples from 142 children newly diagnosed with type 1 diabetes, they found that each of the children had antibodies that were primed to attack cow's milk proteins. These antibodies had apparently arisen in response to cow proteins in their infant formula, but the antibodies were also capable of attacking the body's insulin-producing cells.[4] It turned out that a portion of the cow's milk protein was biochemically an exact match for a portion of human insulin-producing cells. The antibodies that arose to destroy the cow's milk protein ended up attacking the children's insulin-producing cells. The pancreatic cells were destroyed by 'friendly fire'.

This study and others suggested a scenario that could lead to type 1 diabetes: when a very young infant is fed cow's milk formula, some of the milk proteins pass from the digestive tract into the bloodstream.[5,6]

The infant's immune system recognizes these bovine proteins as foreign and forms antibodies to attack them. Unfortunately, these antibodies attack not only the cow proteins but also the insulin-producing cells of the pancreas. This destructive process is gradual; when nearly all the insulin-producing cells are gone, type 1 diabetes results. The researchers believed that the mature digestive tracts of adults would not allow these dairy proteins to pass through the intestinal wall and into the bloodstream, but in infants, the molecules passed through more easily.

The study suggested that one way to prevent type 1 diabetes, at least for many children, might be to avoid exposure to cow's milk early in life. Needless to say, in the early 1990s, neither parents nor paediatricians had any idea about this. Cow's milk formulas were routinely fed to infants, and they still are. When children are not breastfed, some sort of formula has to be used. And while some children are given soya formulas that would presumably pose no diabetes risk, many are given cow's milk varieties.

In 1992, when the *New England Journal of Medicine* report emerged, the well-known paediatrician Dr Benjamin Spock and I held a press conference. We were joined by Dr Frank Oski, director of paediatrics at Johns Hopkins University, and other nutrition experts. We recommended that parents be given information about the potential risks of early exposure to cow's milk. After all, parents are pushed very hard to give milk to their children, but they rarely hear of potential risks it might pose. We called for an end to recommendations that push milk consumption on children and said that parents should have good information in order to decide what to feed their children.

The event proved controversial. Most major newspapers and broadcast channels covered the story. The American Medical Association (AMA) sharply criticized Dr Spock and me for casting doubt on the healthfulness of dairy products. Research teams trying to replicate these findings got mixed results, with some coming up empty-handed. Still other researchers pointed out that finding the antibodies required special techniques, without which the antibodies would remain elusive.[7] Eventually, the American Academy of Pediatrics convened a work group to look into the matter. Two years later, in 1994, the group issued a report. Based on more than 90 studies, the group agreed that indeed, the risk of diabetes can very likely be reduced if infants are not exposed to cow's milk proteins early in life.[8] Eventually, the AMA withdrew its objections.

While Dr Spock and I felt there was already substantial evidence and good reason to issue cautions about exposure to dairy products early in life, the controversy did not end there. There was only one way to know whether dairy proteins could actually incite the series of events leading to type 1 diabetes: the theory had to be put to the test. A European team began that process.

TESTING THE DAIRY-DIABETES THEORY

In a pilot study, researchers in Finland, Sweden and Estonia identified 242 newborns at risk of developing type 1 diabetes – each had a first-degree relative with the condition. The researchers then encouraged their mothers to breastfeed. When mothers were ready to wean their infants, the researchers asked half to use a specially modified baby formula in which dairy proteins were broken up into individual amino acids – protein building blocks that are too small to elicit an immune reaction. The other families were allowed to use a regular cow's milk formula. The research aimed to see whether avoiding exposure to intact cow's milk proteins could reduce the likelihood of developing diabetes.[9]

As the years went by, the researchers found that the children who were fed the special formula were much less likely to develop the dangerous antibodies. In fact, the risk of developing antibodies to their insulin-producing cells was cut by 62 per cent.

The study was small, only a pilot trial, but it did follow most of the children through their first 6 to 8 years of life. During those years, several children developed diabetes. Of those receiving unmodified formula, eight developed the disease, and in the modified-formula group, five developed it. As it turned out, two of those five had dropped out of the study right at the start and never actually received the modified formula. That meant that only three children in the modified-formula group developed diabetes, compared to eight in the regular-formula group. The study suggested that the cow's milk theory may well be part of the puzzle, but it was too small to be definitive, and the research team began a much larger test in 2002 involving families in 15 countries.

There were some limitations to this pilot study. First, it restricted dairy consumption only during the first several months of life. It is not clear whether later exposure, say, at 8 or 9 months of age, might put some children at risk as well. After all, it has long been known that very large dairy protein molecules can sometimes pass from the digestive tract into the bloodstream, even in adults. The study did not address whether exposure to dairy proteins could trigger type 1 diabetes in children who are beyond early infancy.

Second, the study did not ask breastfeeding mothers to avoid cow's milk in their own diets. Many breastfeeding women notice that their children are sometimes affected by what they – the mothers – have eaten. Specifically, if a mother eats certain foods, her baby becomes colicky – crying inconsolably as if suffering from a bad stomach ache. One of the leading suspect foods is dairy products. When breastfeeding women avoid consuming dairy products, their babies often improve. For some women and their babies, it makes an enormous difference.

In 1991, researchers found that some cow's milk proteins ingested by a nursing mother ended up in her breast milk.[10] They came from her digestive tract, were absorbed into her bloodstream, and found their way into the breast milk. Thus, in order to avoid exposing babies to dairy proteins, it is important to eliminate them not only from infants' diets but also from the diets of their breastfeeding mothers.

One last caution about this study: it did not actually exclude dairy products from the children's diets. Rather, it used a milk product treated to break up the dairy proteins. If anything in milk other than these proteins contributes to the problem, this study would not have been able to detect it. Even so, it was an important step in coming to understand how parts of an infant's diet may lead to diabetes.

The study illuminated other contributors to diabetes, too. Prior evidence had suggested that viral infections may play a role, and indeed, viruses appear to have done so for some infants in the milk study. Specifically, viruses seem to stimulate immune cells, perhaps making them more active against cow's milk proteins than they would normally be. Or, cow's milk proteins may influence the course of viral infections in some way.[11] The idea is that the interplay between cow's milk formula and viruses may put babies at increased risk.

No one knows what the research on milk and type 1 diabetes will ultimately show. If the theory turns out to be correct, it suggests that avoiding cow's milk products, at least during the first several months of life, could greatly reduce the likelihood of developing this disease.

Needless to say, breastfeeding instead of feeding formula poses no risks for children. Quite the opposite: breastfed babies gain many advantages, including better overall health and even a few extra IQ points, compared to their formula-fed counterparts. And the most healthy breastfeeding is done when mothers follow a diet free of foods that can harm their babies.

Other risk factors for diabetes may yet emerge in research studies. And for children who are already in the midst of an antibody attack, researchers are studying means of intervening to try to stop the destruction of their insulin-producing cells.

STAYING HEALTHY

If we are able to prevent diabetes, we will have a very powerful tool at our disposal. For people who already have type 1 diabetes, there are effective steps they can take to help them stay healthy. Keeping blood glucose under control is essential, and stabilizing cholesterol levels and blood pressure protects the heart and blood vessels. The same sort of diet that is described in this book for type 2 diabetes is likely to be enormously beneficial for people with type 1 as well.

PART 2

The Programme

CHAPTER 4

A Powerful New Menu

We are setting our sights on a dramatically better result than previous diets could deliver – a result that's possible through a new approach to eating that I will explain in this chapter. If you have type 2 diabetes, you do not want to cater to insulin resistance; you want to counteract it. If you have type 1 diabetes, you want to get your blood sugar under good control, minimize your medications and stay in good health. This chapter will show you the principles of revolutionizing your menu. Then, in the following chapters, I will show you how to put them to work as you plan your meals.

For type 2 diabetes, our goal is to 'clean the gum out of the locks'. As you recall, the fundamental problem in type 2 diabetes appears to be the accumulation of tiny amounts of fat inside muscle cells. They make it hard for insulin to do its job by blocking what is called insulin signalling. That is, they interfere with the process by which insulin opens the cell membrane to allow glucose to enter. You need to select foods that reverse this process.

A diet revamp can also help protect your body from the disease process. That is crucial for both type 1 and type 2 diabetes.

As you will see, these diet changes are far-reaching and powerful. You may also find, as many of our study participants did, that learning the plan's guidelines is a simple process. There are no limits on portions, calories or carbohydrates. You will focus on *what you eat*, so *how much you eat* generally takes care of itself. But we are getting ahead of ourselves.

Let's first look at the menu changes that make the diet so effective. Then, in the following chapter, I will take you through various ways to adopt them to make this diet doable for you.

To reverse the course of diabetes, 'clean the gum out of the locks', and allow the heart and blood vessels the best chance of reversing any existing blockages, there are three guidelines.

1. Set aside animal products.

2. Keep vegetable oils to a minimum.

3. Favour foods with a low glycaemic index.

Now, there is no need to panic. I know this sounds like a tall order. I am going to take you through each step to show you the whys and hows. For now, I just want you to understand the principles.

1. SET ASIDE ANIMAL PRODUCTS

There are two possible sources of fat in the diet: animal products and vegetable oils. This guideline tackles the first of these.

Needless to say, if you are not eating beef, you will not get any beef fat. If you are not eating chicken, you will not get any chicken fat. Following this guideline means purging the animal fat from your diet. The programme you are about to start omits meat, dairy products and eggs.

As you saw in Chapter 2, researchers who measured the fat inside the muscle cells of people on high-fat diets showed that the fat you eat can rapidly increase the amount of fat in your cells. Exactly the opposite happens in people who avoid animal products. As you recall, people following a vegan diet had 31 per cent less intracellular fat compared with people on a regular diet.[1] That means improved insulin sensitivity. That is a great start, and the next guidelines are designed to carry you further.

You will get another benefit. When you set aside animal products, you do more than free yourself from animal fat; since animal products are the only source of cholesterol in the diet, leaving them off your plate also eliminates all the cholesterol from your diet. As your cells reclaim their health, the rest of your body does, too.

Instead of eggs and bacon for breakfast, you might have a big bowl

of old-fashioned porridge with cinnamon or blueberries, half a cantaloupe melon and some rye toast. Perhaps you might add some veggie
sausage or veggie bacon.

For lunch, instead of, say, meat chilli, you might have veggie chilli
or hearty lentil soup. If you generally go for a burger, you might choose
a veggie burger. If you have dinner at an Italian restaurant, you might
have spaghetti with tomato sauce and fresh basil. At a Mexican restaurant, you would skip the meat taco in favour of a bean burrito (without
the cheese). At a Chinese restaurant, you could have your pick of the
many vegetable dishes on a bed of rice.

At this point, you may be thinking, 'Spaghetti? Rice? Am I allowed
to have these carbohydrate-rich foods?' The answer is yes. Now, I
know that people with diabetes have heard over and over that they

Ready for a Change

In our most recent research study, half the volunteers were assigned a low-fat
vegan diet and the other half were instructed to follow a diet based on American
Diabetes Association (ADA) guidelines. Since it was to be an unbiased test, the
diet assignment was done by a computer. The process was random and neither
the volunteers nor we had any influence over who got which diet. Nonetheless, I
was curious about how the volunteers felt about the two diets, so I asked them.
If there had been an opportunity to choose one of the diets, which one would they
have chosen? I expected most to say they would have chosen the ADA diet – it is
familiar to most people who have been diagnosed with diabetes, and I thought
the volunteers might feel a bit of trepidation about giving up meat and dairy
products.

As it turned out, their preferences were just the opposite. *The volunteers actually preferred the vegan diet by about two to one.* The reason, I learned, was that
many of them had already been on the ADA diet and found it dull and not very
effective. Many of them had heard about the advantages of a vegan diet. Others
had relatives who followed a vegetarian or vegan diet, and they wanted to give it
a try.

Both groups embraced their assignments, and as you have read, some did well
on the ADA diet, and some did not. The results with the vegan diet, however,
were powerful and consistent.

must limit rice, pasta and other starchy foods. But keep in mind that diabetes – and overweight – has been rare in countries that have made these foods their staples. The plan does have rules about carbohydrates, but they relate mainly to which ones you choose, not how much. In our studies, we have found that people who include plenty of healthy carbohydrates in their diets do *better*, not worse.

'I can understand omitting beef,' you may say, 'but why eliminate chicken and fish?' Well, the nutritional makeup of these foods may surprise you. They have significant amounts of fat and cholesterol, and they lack the fibre and healthy carbohydrate you need.

Chicken, of course, is where chicken fat comes from. Even if you strip away the skin and eat only white meat, about 23 per cent of the calories come from fat. Much of that fat is the 'bad' form – *saturated* fat, the kind that pushes your cholesterol upwards and worsens insulin resistance.

Fish vary. Some types are lower in fat than chicken, while others, such as salmon, are quite high. But all fish have fat and much of it – between 15 and 30 per cent – is saturated fat. All fish have cholesterol, too. Some, such as prawns and lobster, are much higher in cholesterol, ounce for ounce, than steak.

What a Difference: Animal versus Plant Foods					
ANIMAL FOODS*			PLANT FOODS		
	FAT (% OF CALORIES)	CHOLESTEROL (MG)		FAT (% OF CALORIES)	CHOLESTEROL (MG)
Beef, lean	37	86	Beans, haricot	4	0
Chicken, white meat, skinless	23	85	Broccoli	11	0
Pork loin, lean	41	81	Lentils	3	0
Salmon, Atlantic	40	71	Apple	3	0
Trout, rainbow	35	69	Orange	4	0
Tuna, white	21	42	Rice, brown	7	0

*Meat servings are 100 grams (3.5 ounces).

SOURCE: USDA, Agricultural Research Service Nutrient Data Laboratory, www.nal.usda.gov/fnic/foodcomp/search/index.html, accessed April 7, 2006.

Of course, some people eat fish precisely *because* it has fat in it. That is, a portion of the fat in fish is in the omega-3 form. Omega-3 fats are reputed to reduce inflammation and block the formation of blood clots that could lead to heart attacks. There is increasing evidence, however, that omega-3s are no panacea. In a recent *British Medical Journal* article, a team of British researchers reported the results of a meta-analysis – that is, a large study combining all the prior studies on omega-3s and health. Looking at 89 prior studies, the researchers found that whether omega-3 oils were consumed in fish or as supplements, they offered no significant protection against cardiovascular disease, cancer or risk of death.[2]

Could the supposed benefits of omega-3s be just a fishy tale? Well, it is important to remember that fish fats are mixtures, just as all fats are. Fish oils do indeed contain some omega-3 fat, but they also contain plenty of saturated fat. As noted above, from 15 to 30 per cent of the fat in fish is plain old saturated fat. That's less than in beef (about 50 per cent) or chicken (about 30 per cent), but it is considerably more than you need. There is no specific need for saturated fat in your diet at all.

Finally, if you are looking to lose weight, it is important to note that 'good fats' pack in just as many calories as 'bad fats'. That is to say, omega-3s are every bit as fattening as any other fat or oil.

In studies, chicken-and-fish diets are routinely disappointing. When researchers test diets that include even modest amounts of chicken and fish for their effect on cholesterol, they find that these foods reduce 'bad' low-density lipoprotein (LDL) cholesterol by only about 5 per cent compared to an unrestricted diet.[3] LDL cholesterol is the kind that increases the risk of heart problems.

Much more effective are diets that eliminate animal products altogether. Our most recent study using this sort of diet cut LDL cholesterol by more than 20 per cent. That's four times better than the chicken-and-fish approach.

Now, you will notice that the diet I recommend is not just free of animal fat; it is also free of animal *protein*. That is important because animal protein can harm the kidneys, and protecting them is a key goal. Protein from plant sources is the way to go.

If life without chicken or cheese sounds challenging, take heart from the experiences of the people who participated in our research. They found the transition to be smooth, and within a few weeks they were very much in charge – not only of their menus but also of their health. They found that excess weight was already starting to melt away, their blood sugar was coming under control, their cholesterol levels were falling and, very soon, many started to cut back on – or even discontinue – their medications.

How Nancy and Vance Did It

How did Nancy and Vance, whom you met in the Introduction, fare with the diet changes?

For Nancy, the change was a welcome one. She was fed up with the lack of results from the American Diabetes Association diet and thought a vegetarian diet sounded like a good approach. She wanted to lose weight and she was sick of feeling so low on energy. This, she hoped, might be an answer.

Nancy's mother was not an especially talented cook, she says, but her Scandinavian family loved food. Her mother and sisters all struggled with weight problems.

Like most of our study volunteers, Nancy had already made healthy changes to her diet over the years. She had stopped eating beef, ate plenty of vegetables and had gotten away from fatty dressings, so making the shift was reasonably easy.

She started her day with oats topped with cinnamon and fat-free vanilla soya milk. At midmorning, she liked to have a snack, usually fruit such as apples, bananas, raspberries, blueberries, grapes or oranges.

For lunch, she had a hearty vegan soup such as minestrone, vegetable soup, sweet potato soup or chilli, along with a salad made with spinach leaves; tomatoes; red, yellow and orange peppers; kidney beans and chickpeas; and other ingredients. Her afternoon snack was often fruit, rye crackers, baked tortilla chips with salsa, or hummus and pitta bread.

After a long day at work, Nancy had no interest in preparing a gourmet meal, so her dinners were quick and easy: a veggie burger with frozen mixed vegetables, which she microwaved. Sometimes she had nothing more than a bowl of bran cereal. A late-night fruit snack rounded things off.

We gave her group a supermarket tour and provided cooking demonstrations to introduce everyone to healthy products that might be new to them. Nancy preferred to keep it simple and started making a large pot of soup to eat all week. 'I am not a cook,' she said. 'And I find it very easy to stay on this programme.'

Vance usually started his day with oats, either plain or with apples and cinnamon. He also had toast and fresh fruit. Lunch or dinner was pasta or burritos along with fresh vegetables and fruits. Sometimes his taste called for salads, usually dressed up with beans, blood oranges or other additions.

'I had to learn to read labels,' he said. 'It is easy to underestimate the amount of fat or sugar in a can of food. A label might show 6 grams of fat, and you might think that means the whole can. But it actually means just one serving.'

For Vance, the vegan diet was the way to go. 'I don't have the personality that would let me have just a small piece of chicken or a small piece of beef,' he explained. 'I have to cut it out altogether. For me, this is a lifestyle change.'

Healthier Substitutes for Dairy Products

It may surprise you to learn that some of the biggest sources of fat are lurking in the dairy section. Milk, cheese and ice cream once enjoyed a healthy reputation that few people questioned, but that has changed. It has become clear that these foods contribute not only fat but also cholesterol, animal protein and, in the case of fat-free varieties, a big load of lactose sugar.

Soup Nirvana

Walter arrived at one of our research meetings to announce that he had found the perfect lunch. His local supermarket stocks a line of soups that happen to come in several low-fat vegan varieties, such as mixed bean soup and split pea soup.

Soups are a great source of quick, simple meals for vegans as they come in a wide variety of flavours. Look for brands that have just a gram or two of fat per serving. One brand to look out for is Amy's, which has a range of tasty low-fat soups suitable for vegans. It's a US brand but is becoming more readily available in other countries.

Nutrition Guidelines

Here is a simple summary of the guidelines presented in this chapter. You should follow them exactly, because even slight variations may affect your results.

Overall Principles

Choose foods from plant sources. Avoid all animal products and keep vegetable oils to a bare minimum. Favour foods with a low glycaemic index (GI).

Focus on the New Four Food Groups

Whole Grains: Whole grain pasta, brown rice, bran cereal, oats, pumpernickel or rye bread, couscous, bulgur wheat, millet, barley, etc. Suggested servings: 8 per day. One serving is 75 g (2½ oz) cooked grain (e.g., oats or pasta), 30 g (1 oz) dry cereal, or 1 slice bread.

Pulses: Beans (black or kidney beans; chickpeas; baked beans; soyabeans, etc.), peas, split peas, lentils, low-fat soya products (unsweetened soya milk, low-fat veggie burgers, textured vegetable protein, low-fat tofu), etc. Suggested servings: 3 per day. One serving is 75 g (2½ oz) cooked beans, 115 g (4 oz) tofu or 240 ml (8 fl oz) soya milk.

Vegetables: Sweet potatoes, broccoli, cauliflower, spinach, kale, squash, green beans, pak choi, artichokes, etc. Choose those with a low GI. Suggested servings: 4 or more per day. A serving is 125 g (4½ oz) raw or 75 g (2½ oz) cooked vegetables.

Fruits: Apples, bananas, grapes, pears, peaches, oranges, kiwifruit, berries, etc. Choose those with a low GI. Suggested servings: 3 or more per day. One serving is one piece raw fruit, 75 g (2½ oz) chopped or cooked fruit, or 120 ml (4 fl oz) juice.

Here's the lowdown on dairy, followed by the good news about how easy it is to replace it.

Dairy fat. Cow's milk derives, believe it or not, roughly 49 per cent of its calories from fat. That is a lot by any standard. You may imagine that semi-skimmed milk is much lower in fat. Not so. It is approximately 1.7 per cent fat – a figure that refers to fat content *by weight*, which is deceptive because it is thrown off by milk's water content. When you drink a glass of milk, your body absorbs that water. What matters for your health is how much fat you are left with. Nutritionists look for the *percentage of calories* that come from fat because that figure

Other Permitted Foods

- Fat-free salad dressings and other fat-free condiments

- Coffee, tea (with fat-free nondairy creamer, if desired)

- Occasionally, alcoholic beverages

- Rarely, sugar, nuts, seeds, dark chocolate (made without milk), full-fat soya products such as tofu, tempeh, soya cheese, etc.

Foods to Avoid

- Meats, poultry, fish, eggs (whites and yolks) and all dairy products (regular and fat-free), including milk, yogurt, cheese, ice cream, cream, soured cream, butter, etc.

- Added oils, such as margarine, salad dressings, mayonnaise, cooking oils, etc.

- Fried foods, such as potato crisps, french fries, onion rings, doughnuts, etc.

- Avocados, olives and peanut butter

- Refined foods and/or foods with a high glycaemic index, such as white bread and white potatoes

A Daily Multivitamin

Take a daily multivitamin as a convenient source of vitamin B_{12} (unless you choose B_{12}-fortified products such as fortified breakfast cereals or fortified soya milk) and vitamin D, which you may need if you rarely get exposure to natural sunlight.

is unaffected by water content. It turns out that for semi-skimmed milk, about 31 per cent of calories come from nothing but fat.

What is particularly worrisome about milk, though, is the *type* of fat it contains. Most of it is saturated fat, the very kind that is linked to insulin resistance and raises cholesterol levels.

Typical yogurt, ice cream and soured cream products are high in fat, too. Cheese is loaded with it. Many brands derive about 70 per cent of their calories from fat.

Dairy sugar. Fat-free dairy products have had their fat removed, but what's still there may surprise you. When the fat is skimmed away, the predominant nutrient in milk is actually sugar – lactose, the dairy sugar.

The lactose molecule is a combination of two smaller sugars, glucose and galactose. Approximately 55 per cent of the calories in fat-free milk come from lactose. People who quite rightly avoid fizzy drinks because of their sugar content will want to be aware that milk products are a major source of sugar, too.

Lactose, of course, is the sugar that causes digestive upset for many people. Lactose intolerance is a normal condition that occurs when the enzymes that allow babies to digest mother's milk naturally start to dissipate. When these enzymes are gone, lactose passes through the intestinal tract undigested. In the lower intestinal tract, bacteria start to ferment the sugar, causing wind, cramps and diarrhoea. Lactose intolerance was once thought to be an abnormality but is now known to be the biological norm. The symptoms come on gradually, sometime after early childhood, and they are simply a sign that you have successfully passed the age of weaning.

Dairy proteins. These proteins have come under scrutiny for their potential contribution to type 1 diabetes, as described in Chapter 3, but they are implicated in many other health concerns as well. Animal proteins appear to accelerate the gradual loss of kidney function that can occur in diabetes.[4] Plant sources of protein – beans, grains, vegetables and soya products, for example – do not appear to cause this problem.

People who have migraines often report improvement when they avoid certain foods, and milk and other dairy products are often at the top of the list. The same has been reported for some cases of rheumatoid arthritis. The problem, it appears, is not the fat or lactose, at least not for these conditions. The trigger seems to be the dairy proteins.

Dairy products are linked to other health problems ranging from acne to prostate and ovarian cancer. It is the latter issue – cancer – that has gotten the attention of the medical community. Two large Harvard studies and several other studies from other countries have shown that milk-drinking men have a significantly higher risk of prostate cancer compared with men who generally avoid milk.[5,6] The explanation appears to lie in hormonal effects caused by milk. For ovarian cancer, the evidence is mixed, with some studies showing higher risk among milk drinkers and others showing no increased risk.[7,8]

Milk's selling point has been the calcium it provides. There are, however, better calcium sources and more effective ways of maintaining strong bones. I will go into more detail about this later in the chapter.

Making better choices. People who avoid dairy products find no shortage of great substitutes. Health food stores and supermarkets stock soya milk, rice milk, almond milk and many others. They come in regular, calcium-fortified and low-fat varieties and in plain vanilla, chocolate and strawberry flavours. You will want to choose those lowest in fat and sugar. Calcium-fortified juices have arrived on the market, too. Of course, none of these is necessary. After the age of weaning, the only beverage that is actually biologically required is water. Not juice, not milk – just pure water.

There are many delicious nondairy ice cream substitutes made from soya or rice milk. In many cases, however, the main reason they are so delicious is that they contain added sugar. Your taste buds can be easily seduced by these treats, but your body would be far better off with a bowl of strawberries.

Alternatives to Eggs

There are just two problems with eggs: the yolk and the white. The yolk is where cholesterol lurks, with 213 milligrams in a single egg. That's more than in an 8-ounce steak.

The yolk also holds the fat, about 5 grams per egg. Egg white has problems of its own, since it is essentially pure animal protein. As you know by now, animal protein can present problems for your kidneys, and you are better off with plant protein.

Can there really be all that fat, cholesterol and animal protein inside a single egg? Certainly. Keep in mind that when an egg hatches, a baby chick emerges. That chick's body was formed from what was inside the egg when it was laid. Like all animal products, eggs have no fibre at all and no complex carbohydrate.

There are plenty of great ways to replace eggs, whether you are hooked on scrambled eggs for breakfast or baked goods that include eggs. Try these substitutes.

- If a recipe calls for just 1 or 2 eggs, leave them out. Add a couple of extra tablespoons of water for moisture.

- Egg replacement powders are available in many health food stores.

- Use 1 heaped tablespoon soya flour or cornflour plus 2 tablespoons water to replace each egg in baked products.

- Try an egg-size piece of mashed tofu in place of each egg.

- Half a mashed banana can be used in muffin and cookie recipes, although it will provide its own flavour.

- For meatless loaves and veggie burgers, use any of the following to bind the ingredients together: tomato purée, mashed potato, moistened breadcrumbs or rolled oats.

For a breakfast dish to replace scrambled eggs, scrambled tofu has become popular. When you see the Menus and Recipes section, you will discover why. Tofu has a texture very much like egg white and takes on the flavour of whatever it is cooked with. Be wary of products promoted as no-cholesterol egg replacements; many are simply egg whites with various added ingredients.

2. KEEP VEGETABLE OILS TO A MINIMUM

Oils creep in everywhere, it seems: cooking oils, salad oils, vegetable oils used in baking and in snack foods. Vegetable oils do enjoy a better reputation than animal fat, and indeed, they have less saturated fat – the kind that raises cholesterol levels. But we still want to keep *all* oils to a minimum. Here is why.

First, as you know by now, all fats and oils are loaded with calories. They have 9 calories per gram, which is more than twice the calorie content of carbohydrate or protein (4 calories per gram). Thus, when it comes to calorie content, vegetable oils are as fattening as lard. All fats and oils are in fact equally fattening.

Second, if your goal is to regain as much insulin sensitivity as possible, you will want to eliminate not only animal fats but also added vegetable oils. Cleaning the animal fat out of your cellular 'locks' does no good if you are going to clog them with vegetable grease. Here are the sources of these oils.

Fried foods. French fries, potato crisps, onion rings and other fried snacks are essentially sponges carrying grease from the deep fryer to your body fat stores.

Added oils. Typical salad dressings and margarines have lots of fat.

Oils used as ingredients. Many packaged foods and sauces include significant amounts of oil.

Oils used in sautéing. Many recipes begin with the instruction to sauté onions, garlic or other ingredients in oil. Some restaurants use oil almost as a staple.

There are easy ways to avoid all that grease.

- Steer clear of fried snacks such as potato crisps and french fries.

- Top salads with fat-free dressings, lemon juice or balsamic vinegar.

- Use nonstick pans.

- Steam-fry onions, garlic or vegetables in water or another cooking liquid instead of sautéing the traditional way. See the Menus and Recipes section.

- Steam vegetables.

- Consider using cooking spray to dispense small traces of oil in place of poured oils.

- Use fat-free nondairy coffee creamer.

- Read food labels. Look for products with no more than 2 to 3 grams of fat per serving or with a percentage of calories from fat of below 10 per cent.

When it comes to avoiding greasy foods, some people are eager to make an exception for olive oil. It seems natural and even chic. But think for a second about how factories manage to fill a bottle with oil. They take an enormous number of olives, discard their fibre and pulp, and leave you with pure fat.

Gram for gram, olive oil has the same number of calories as beef fat, chicken fat and other fats and oils – that is, 9 calories per gram. No other food is more calorie dense. While olive oil contains a great deal of monounsaturated fat, which has little or no effect on cholesterol, it also contains saturated fat (about 13 per cent), the kind that increases cholesterol and worsens insulin resistance. It does not matter how expensive the oil is or how 'extra virgin' it may be. It still has more calories and saturated fat than your body is designed to process to maintain optimal health.

There are, of course, traces of natural vegetable oils in vegetables, fruits, beans and grains, but you need not worry about them. Your body does need a tiny amount of fat, and plants provide it naturally. We run into problems when oils are concentrated, as they are in fried foods, oily sauces and recipes with added oils.

A few plant foods, such as nuts, seeds, olives, avocados and some soya products, are naturally high in oil. You will want to keep them to a minimum.

What About Good Fats?

There are two types of fat your body actually needs. Their technical names are alpha-linolenic acid and linoleic acid. These terms are not important; you will never see them on an ingredients list. What is important to know is that you only need a tiny amount of them. The body's need for these essential fats is no more than 2 to 3 per cent of your daily calorie intake.

Where do you find them? Beans, vegetables and fruits are very low in fat overall, but the traces they do contain are relatively rich in 'good' fat – that is, alpha-linolenic acid. This is the basic omega-3 fat that your body uses to produce other good fats. Nuts, seeds and soya products contain larger amounts. Linoleic acid is found in many plant foods, too.

Some people boost the omega-3 fats in their diets to treat arthritis, for example. If you are doing this, be careful: all fats, good and bad, are equally fattening, and many contain things your body does not need. Fish oil, for example, contains plenty of saturated fat along with its omega-3s. At the end of this chapter, I will describe more healthy omega-3 sources.

The best way to get the right kind and amount of fat in your diet is to skip animal products, fried foods and oily food products and get your nutrition from vegetables, fruits, beans and whole grains.

Does it really matter whether or not we avoid animal products and added oils? Absolutely. A typical European or North American diet might provide 80 to 100 grams of fat per day, or even more. Switching from beef to chicken and fish, keeping portions modest and limiting added oils will trim this to about 60 grams. But setting animal products aside and avoiding added oils can drop this number to close to 20 grams. In the process, your cholesterol intake, which would be well over 200 milligrams per day on an unmodified diet, will drop to zero. Zero! Every cell in your body will thank you.

3. FAVOUR FOODS WITH A LOW GLYCAEMIC INDEX

You will find this third guideline very useful. The glycaemic index (GI) is a handy tool that was invented by David Jenkins, MD, PhD, DSc, a physician and researcher at the University of Toronto.[9] It is simply a number that indicates how rapidly any given food releases sugar into the bloodstream. A food with a high GI releases sugar into the blood quickly.

One example is white bread. If the molecules of carbohydrate in bread were greatly magnified, they would look like strings of beads. Each bead is a molecule of sugar (glucose). In your digestive tract, these beads separate and pass into your bloodstream.

With white bread, this process is quick. The string of beads rapidly disintegrates and the individual glucose molecules race into your bloodstream. If you were to check your blood sugar after eating the bread, you would see the result. White bread has a high GI, meaning it has a pronounced effect on your blood glucose.

In contrast, pumpernickel bread has a low GI.* Its string of beads comes apart more slowly, passing into the bloodstream bit by bit. It has much less effect on your blood sugar.

In a nutshell, high-GI foods tend to have a greater effect on your blood sugar, and low-GI foods have less effect.

I should mention that when researchers measure the GI of individual foods, they test volunteers who do not have diabetes, so a food that does not raise their blood sugar very much could raise yours somewhat more. However, the point of the glycaemic index is to allow us to rate foods – to compare one against another – so we can choose the best ones.

---

*The glycaemic index of a food is determined by feeding a portion containing 50 grams of carbohydrate to 10 healthy people after an overnight fast. Blood glucose is tested at 15- to 30-minute intervals over the next 2 hours, and the result is compared to that of feeding the same amount of glucose (or in some cases, white bread). A GI below 100 means the test food has less effect on blood sugar than glucose. A higher number means the food has a greater effect.[10]

On page 56, you will find a table of the GI values of many common foods. Let me first summarize a few easy things to look for so you can size up most foods without consulting a table.

Glycaemic Index at a Glance

- Beans and their relatives (lentils, peas) are always low GI.

- Green leafy vegetables can also be considered low GI (although they have so little starch that their GIs typically have not been calculated).

- Nearly all fruits have a low GI. Yes, they are sweet, but most will not raise your blood sugar terribly quickly. Two exceptions: watermelon and pineapple have a higher GI than other fruits.

- Pasta is a low-GI food. Surprising, but true.

- Barley, bulgur and parboiled/converted rice (such as Uncle Ben's) all have a low GI value.

- Pumpernickel and rye breads have a lower GI value, while wheat varieties such as bagels, white bread and even wholemeal bread have a higher GI.

- Yams and sweet potatoes are low-GI foods in contrast to baking potatoes, which have a high GI.

- Among breakfast cereals, oats and bran cereals have a lower GI, while most cold cereals tend to have a high GI.

Now, if you have type 2 diabetes, *any* food with carbohydrate in it will push your blood sugar up to a degree. In fact, a rise in blood glucose after a meal is normal, and if your cells are insulin resistant, it takes a bit more time for glucose in your bloodstream to pass into your cells. This does not mean, however, that you should avoid foods that contain carbohydrate. What it means is that you will want to take steps to reduce your insulin resistance, as outlined in this chapter. Among carbohydrates, the best are those with a low GI.

The reason I mention this is that sometimes people with type 2 diabetes shun carbohydrates. They avoid rice, beans, pasta and all the rest and load up on chicken, fish and eggs because these foods have no carbohydrate. But over the long run, they find their blood sugar does not improve; their level gets worse, so they need more and more medicine.

It makes sense when you think about the accumulation of fat in cells – more gum in the locks, so to speak. Greasy meals today mean insulin resistance tomorrow.

It may surprise you to learn that pasta has a low GI. It does, particularly if it is served *al dente*, that is, not overcooked. Of course, pasta is made from wheat flour, so you may think it would spike your blood sugar in the same way as wheat bread. But that is not the case.

Pasta actually gives us a little lesson in why some foods have a high GI, while the GI of others is low.

Let's say we are making bread dough. We add a bit of yeast to the flour to make the bread rise. The yeast causes many tiny air pockets to form, which is what makes bread different from, say, a shingle. Now, as you eat the baked bread, your stomach acid and digestive enzymes enter those air pockets and rapidly break the molecules of flour into individual sugar molecules that then pass from your digestive tract into your bloodstream. Even wholemeal bread, with shreds of fibre remaining, is easy pickings for digestive enzymes – they have no difficulty entering the air pockets and digesting the starch in the bread.

Pasta is different. It is not made with yeast, so it has no air pockets. If bread is like a pile of tiny twigs, ready to ignite with a single spark, pasta is like a cord of logs – it is much more compacted and 'catches fire' more slowly. Even if you chew pasta thoroughly, there is no way it can digest as rapidly as bread – and that's why it has a lower GI.

The simple lesson is that processing foods – pulverizing grains into flour or using yeast to make dough rise, for example – starts the digestive process before you even put the food on your plate. An intact grain is slow to come apart and release glucose into your bloodstream, while a heavily processed grain disintegrates quickly. Thus, old-fashioned porridge, which consists of whole oats, has a low GI. But quick-cooking oats are made by slicing the oat grains into fragments. That allows them to cook faster and to digest faster – which means a higher GI.

If you would like to look up the GI of individual foods, you can take a look at a website established at the University of Sydney in Australia: www.glycaemicindex.com. Just type in the name of the food, and all the testing results will appear.

The Glycaemic Index of Common Foods

GRAINS AND GRAIN PRODUCTS	GI	FRUIT	GI
All-Bran cereal	38	Apple	44
Barley, pearled	25	Apricot	57
Bread, pumpernickel	55	Banana	51
Bread, rye	63	Cantaloupe melon	65
Bread, white	70	Grapes	43
Bread, wholemeal	70	Orange	48
Corn	60	Peach	28
Oatmeal, instant	65	Pear	33
Oatmeal, old-fashioned	62	Pineapple	66
Quinoa	53	Raisins	64
Rice, brown	50	Strawberries	40
Rice, parboiled	48	Watermelon	72
Rice, white	72	**VEGETABLES**	**GI**
Spaghetti	48	Beetroot	64
PULSES	**GI**	Carrot	41
Beans, kidney	29	Parsnip	97
Beans, haricot	39	Potato, new	70
Chickpeas	36	Potato, russet, baked	94
Lentils, red	31	Sweet potato	48
Peas	22	Yam	51

Notes: Values of 55 or below are considered low, 56 to 69 are medium, and 70 and above are high.

Values should be considered approximations only. Many of these foods have been tested in various countries under varying conditions. Listings represent typical, not exact, values.

GI values are calculated only for foods containing sugar or starch. Certain foods, such as broccoli, cauliflower and many berries, are high in fibre but very low in starch, so a GI value cannot be calculated. Similarly, avocados are high in fat and low in starch and consequently do not have a GI.

SOURCE: www.glycaemicindex.com, accessed April 8, 2006.

'Does it really matter?' you may be asking. 'Can it really make a difference if my porridge is old-fashioned instead of instant, or if I introduce beans, green leafy vegetables and barley soups into my diet?' Jennie Brand-Miller, PhD, of the University of Sydney, answered that question by analysing the combined results of 14 studies on the glycaemic index that included a total of 356 participants. She found that choosing low-GI foods reduces HbA1c by 0.3 to 0.4 percentage point. In some studies, the difference was as much as 0.6 point.[11] Studies showed a similar benefit for both type 1 and type 2 diabetes.

This advantage is over and above that of the other diet changes you are making. As you will remember from Chapter 2, the combined diet changes described in this book – avoiding animal products, minimizing oils and eating low-GI foods – added up to an HbA1c drop of 1.2 percentage points, on average, in our research. That average includes people who did not have very far to drop as well as some participants who started with HbA1cs in the 9 to 10 per cent range and dropped several percentage points. These results are stronger than any single drug is likely to bring. For some people, that is all it takes to return their HbA1c to the normal range.

PUTTING THE RIGHT FUEL IN YOUR TANK

Now we have covered the basics, the three guidelines that work together to help you regain control: avoiding animal products, keeping oils to a minimum and favouring low-GI foods.

These guidelines work together. Meeting one of them is not enough. For example, jelly beans can be vegan and they are low in oil. Because they are essentially solid sugar, though, they have a high GI and will spike your blood glucose.

Similarly, a piece of cake loaded with butter can have a very low GI because butter contains no carbohydrate and may even slow the absorption of glucose you eat. But the cake is not vegan, nor is it low in fat. It will contribute to insulin resistance, and you want to steer clear of it. The low GI is not a reason to eat it if it does not meet our other criteria.

The three guidelines together are a powerful combination. Nancy's HbA1c was 8.3 per cent at the beginning of our study. As she began the healthy diet changes, it rapidly slid under 7.0, even while she reduced her medications. For Vance, initial HbA1c testing showed a value of 9.5 per cent, but as the weeks went by, it dropped and dropped and dropped. By the study's conclusion, his HbA1c was a healthy 5.3 per cent.

Now, before we plan out your breakfast, lunch and dinner, let me show you how these three principles translate into changes inside your body. Just as a car performs dramatically better when it has the fuel it was designed for, your body performs far better when you give it the foods it needs.

Increased insulin sensitivity. As you know by now, evidence shows that a diet change can have a quick and decisive influence on the amount of fat inside your cells. As the amount of fat drops, your cells become more and more sensitive to insulin, allowing your blood sugar to come down. If your insulin resistance was previously worsening and your medication doses increasing, the process begins to reverse.

This can happen remarkably quickly. In fact, it can happen so quickly that I need to encourage you, if you are using insulin or any drug that increases insulin secretion (for example, glipizide, glimepiride, nateglinide, repaglinide, rosiglitazone or glibenclamide*), to be in close touch with your doctor. As your cells regain their insulin sensitivity, you will become more and more like a healthy person who is taking drugs they no longer need.

The combination of a good diet and the drugs you have been taking can drive your blood sugar down to healthy levels and then below them, to hypoglycaemia. Your doctor will lower your medication doses or even discontinue your medications as necessary. Now, do not throw your medicines away on your own. The process is gradual, and your doctor will guide you. And do not be frightened by this return to health. It is a wonderful feeling to discover that your insulin sensitivity is improving day by day. When your doctor says it's time to cut back on medication or stop a drug altogether, it is as if time is moving backwards.

Chapter 7 has important details on how to prevent and treat hypoglycaemic episodes. Please read it carefully before changing your diet.

Easy weight control. If you have been hoping to lose weight, that process has just begun. On average, the diet you are beginning causes a weight loss of about 0.5 kg (1 lb) per week. As time goes on, it adds up to an impressive change.

'How does this work?' you may ask. How can you lose weight if you are paying no attention at all to portion sizes, calories and carbohydrates? There are three main reasons.

---

*UK trade names are Glibenese, Minodiab (glipizide); Amaryl (glimepiride); Starlix (nateglinide); Avandia (rosiglitazone); Avandamet (a combination of metformin and rosiglitazone); Novonorm (repaglinide); and Daonil, Euglucon (glibenclamide).

First, the foods have very little fat, so you are eliminating the main source of unwanted calories.

Second, the vegetables, fruits, beans and whole grains you are introducing into your diet give you a healthy dose of fibre, which is filling enough to turn off your appetite a bit sooner than would happen without them. On average, each 14 grams of fibre cuts about 10 per cent off your calorie intake. A person who normally eats 2,000 calories per day and then starts to add an extra 14 grams of fibre daily will tend to feel full after eating 1,800 calories.[12]

Third, these foods cause a slight boost in your after-meal calorie burn. Normally, you burn calories faster after a meal due to the processes of digestion. Our studies have shown that a low-fat vegan diet increases this after-meal burn, giving you an extra edge.[13] I will go over this in more detail in Chapter 6. For now, just enjoy the weight control that is kicking in on its own.

Losing excess weight feels great, of course, but weight loss improves your insulin sensitivity in addition to the effects of the diet change itself.

Easy cholesterol control. If you have had a cholesterol problem, the programme you are now beginning is far more powerful than typical cholesterol-lowering diets. This should be no surprise. Your new diet is not *low* in cholesterol; it has no cholesterol *at all*. It also has no animal fat, which is important because animal fat (like other sources of saturated fat) encourages your body to make cholesterol. They are all gone now. You have replaced them with cholesterol-lowering oats, soya and other botanical magicians, as you will see in more detail in Chapter 12.

Your arteries are starting to breathe a sigh of relief. The damage of diabetes is done to the arteries, for the most part, leading to problems in your heart, eyes, kidneys and nerves. But now, you are inhibiting that process, and bringing your cholesterol level down is part of it. You are following the kind of diet used in programmes to *reverse* heart disease.

Again, do not throw your medications away and cancel your doctor appointments. Your doctor can size up your heart health and track your progress.

Reversing symptoms. A team of California researchers used a low-fat vegan diet, combined with exercise, in a group of 21 people with type 2 diabetes, all of whom had painful neuropathy – the nerve symptoms that arise as the nerves show signs of damage. In just 2 weeks, 17 of the 21 reported complete cessation of their nerve symptoms, and the remaining 4 had noticeable improvements.[14]

Other researchers have found that some of the changes in the eye – exudates in the retina – that sometimes occur in diabetes start to improve or even disappear when people make a healthy diet change. The loss of protein through the kidneys can also diminish. You will find more details on all of these in Chapter 13.

FIRST STEPS

One of the things we have carefully tested with this programme is how people *feel* about it. Bottom line: although you will be making major changes in your menu that are designed to bring you uncompromised good health, this is perhaps the easiest diet change to stick with over the long run. Partly, that is because it is not a 'diet'. It is a different way of regarding food – a much better way of thinking about and enjoying it. Also, you will never go hungry and never tease yourself with minuscule portions of foods you love.

Let me show you the steps that make it that way. For the moment, you are not actually going to change anything. I just want to take you through the steps that will get you started.

Step 1: Use the New Four Food Groups

For starters, let me introduce you to a basic meal-planning guide that my colleagues and I developed in 1991. It is called the New Four Food Groups, and it is a big improvement on the old four food groups that the United States Department of Agriculture (USDA) developed in 1956 and on the various pyramid-shaped graphics developed since then (these graphics and guidelines were very influential and were taken up by many other countries). The idea is simple: build your diet from four healthy staples – whole grains, pulses, vegetables and fruits.

On your plate, these simple ingredients might translate into a hearty sweet potato soup, spinach lasagne, curried chickpeas and rice, or lentil and carrot soup. And there are endless other possibilities. But let's first take a look at the staple food groups themselves. These are the ingredients that build the most healthy meals.

The whole grain group. This group includes brown rice, oats, barley, corn and all the products that are made from whole grains: breads, cereals, pasta and many others. In countries where grains are staples, diabetes is much less common than it is in Europe and North America. This should be no surprise: whole grains are filling but have very little fat and no cholesterol. When selecting grains, let the glycaemic index guide you.

The pulse group. This category includes beans, peas and lentils. It also includes the endless array of soya products, from veggie burgers to meatless sausages, tofu, tempeh and miso. Pulses are hearty, high-protein foods with a remarkably low GI. They are rich in calcium, iron, cholesterol-lowering soluble fibre, and even traces of 'good' fats – omega-3 fatty acids. Whether you favour a chickpea salad, kidney bean chilli or a soya-based veggie burger or other meat substitute, pulses are handy, healthy ingredients.

The one thing the bean group lacks is good public relations. Its health benefits have gone largely unnoticed. Nutrition scientists, however, know that putting these healthy powerhouses front and centre on your menu is a great way to drive down your weight, blood sugar and cholesterol. Findings from the US government's National Nutrition and Health Examination Survey, conducted from 1999 to 2002, showed that people who included beans in their regular menu weighed, on average, 3 kg (6.5 lb) less than people who generally neglected this healthy food group.[15] The trend showed up in teenagers, too. Teenage bean lovers weighed 3.15 kg (7 lb) less and had waistlines that were nearly 2.5 cm (1 in) slimmer compared with their bean-avoiding peers.[16]

Researchers at the University of Kentucky summarized the results of 11 prior research studies and found that people who frequently consume pulses are indeed thinner. They also have lower levels of 'bad' LDL cholesterol and higher levels of 'good' HDL (high-density lipoprotein) cholesterol.[17]

If you are new to bean dishes, go easy at first, and keep portions modest. They are likely to cause some wind until your digestive tract adapts.

The vegetable group. Each member of the vegetable group is robustly healthy. The green vegetables – asparagus, broccoli, spinach, kale, cabbage and many others – are packed with iron and, except for spinach, high in absorbable calcium. Orange vegetables are loaded with beta–carotene, a cancer fighter. You will get it from carrots, yams and butternut squash, among others. Be generous with them.

Instead of the neglected little pile of overcooked vegetables some people park on their plates, have at least two or even three different vegetables with your dinner. One of my favourite combinations is mashed butternut squash and broccoli. Sometimes I cook them up fresh, and other times, I simply use frozen. The colours contrast, as does the sweetness of the squash with the heartier flavour of broccoli. You do not have to be a gourmet chef to cook vegetables. Even the most hurried person has time to open a packet of frozen vegetables and steam or microwave them.

These foods are loaded with vitamins and minerals, are very low in fat, and like all plant foods, have no cholesterol at all.

Virtually all have a healthy low GI. The main exception is baking potatoes, so favour sweet potatoes and yams instead.

The fruit group. Fruits are loaded with vitamins and of course have no fat or cholesterol. Many people with diabetes imagine that because fruits are sweet, they will raise blood sugar. The fact is, though, that nearly all fruits – apples, bananas, blueberries, cherries, clemen-

Grapefruit Interacts with Medications

Surprising as it sounds, if you are on medications, you may need to avoid grapefruit. This citrus fruit inhibits intestinal enzymes that metabolize several medications.[18] A glass of grapefruit juice can measurably increase the blood concentrations of cholesterol-lowering drugs, such as atorvastatin (Lipitor) and simvastatin (Zocor), among others. It does the same for drugs commonly used to control blood pressure, such as amlodipine (Istin), nifedipine (Adalat, Coracten), and verapamil (Cordilox, Securon). Ditto for antihistamines and some psychiatric medications, such as diazepam (Valium).

The grapefruit effect lasts for 24 hours or more, and in rare cases, the concentrations of drugs in the bloodstream can increase to toxic levels. These lists are not exhaustive, and the effects vary from one person to another, so if you are on any medication, check with your doctor about how grapefruit might affect you. Researchers are currently testing the extent to which other citrus juices, such as orange juice, may have similar effects.

Note: trade names given here are UK trade names.

tines, oranges, peaches, pears and most others – have a low GI. The exceptions are watermelon and pineapple.

How many servings should you have from each group? The chart on page 46 provides some basic guidelines, but you can vary these serving sizes as much as you like. If you prefer Mediterranean cuisine, your plate may be rich in vegetables and pasta. If Oriental food is your thing, your plate may hold generous portions of whole grains. If you love all types of cuisine, you will probably want lots of variety. In the next chapter, I will show you some easy, delicious ways to get started.

It goes without saying that the recommended foods do not include meat, dairy products, eggs or greasy fried foods. You should also add a daily multivitamin. It will provide vitamin B_{12}, which you need for healthy blood and nerves and which is not found in substantial amounts in plant foods, except for fortified products. A multi also provides vitamin D. While sunlight on your skin provides D naturally, modern life takes most of us out of the sun. In choosing a multivitamin, I would suggest an iron-free brand unless your doctor recommends otherwise. Most people have plenty of stored iron already, and iron overload can be harmful.

Okay, now that you understand the New Four Food Groups, at least in theory, let's move on to the next step.

Step 2: Try Out a Recipe or Two

Before you jump into a new way of eating, take a few recipes for a test-drive. Look through the next chapter for ideas and browse through the Menus and Recipes section. You will find a great many possibilities to get you started. If you rarely cook and eat at restaurants often, the next chapter will have many tips on things you can look for.

Your goal is to identify healthy breakfasts, lunches and dinners that you really like. That means meals that meet all of our guidelines (no animal products, minimal vegetable oils and low GI) *and* appeal to your tastes.

Remember that this new way of eating does not mean making a new dish every night. Dr William Castelli, former director of the Framingham Heart Study, used to say that most of us tend to stick to our favourite meals. We may have eight or nine different dinners we

like, and we pick from that repertoire night after night. All you need
to do is to find eight or nine *healthy* meals that suit your tastes, and you
are set.

Step 3: Pick 3 Weeks

Some people like to ease their way gradually into a healthier diet pattern. If you are among that group, go ahead and take your time getting
to know healthier foods. But I advise a different approach. Mark a 3-
week period on your calendar when you plan to embrace this programme. Before you reach your start date, identify meals that fit our
criteria and appeal to you. When the start day arrives, commit yourself
completely for 21 days.

As I tell our research participants, this is not the time to stick your
toe in the swimming pool; it's time to jump in. Really do it. There are
two reasons for this.

First, it gives you fast results. If you have a healthy meal on Monday
and another on Saturday, your body will not notice any difference. But
if you do it at every meal, gains come quickly. Give yourself a chance
to see how it feels to be on as perfect a diet as possible.

The second reason is that a diet change really is like getting into a
swimming pool. If you ease your way into the water bit by bit, it is a
painful process. But if you plunge in, very soon you see that the water
feels fine. Let me explain.

Did you ever switch from whole milk to skimmed milk? If you are
like most people, that first glass of fat-free seemed watery and maybe
even discoloured. After a couple of weeks, though, you became totally
used to the lighter taste. Before long, whole milk seemed thick and
distasteful.

Now, I am not suggesting that skimmed milk is a health food. As
you have seen, there are good reasons to avoid it. But when you lighten
your diet, your tastes rapidly change. Very soon, you come to prefer the
new, healthier taste.

You will find that your taste buds have a memory of about 3 weeks,
and jumping into the diet change allows them to adjust quickly. Instead
of pining over the unhealthy foods you have left behind, you will be
surprised to find that you miss them very little.

If a 100 per cent diet change sounds like a tall order, let me make it a bit more approachable. You do not need to commit to it forever; you just need to give it a try. At this point, there's no need to swear you will never again eat a double cheeseburger, pledge your loyalty to oatmeal or make any other daunting promises. Just give it 3 weeks. During that time, really do it 100 per cent, and you will get a good sense of what the diet will do while still keeping all your options open.

Step 4: Get to Know Transition Foods

Modern technology has brought us plenty of modern annoyances (ringing mobile phones, crowded roads and junk e-mail), but once in a while, it's actually useful. The food industry has managed to mimic unhealthy foods with more healthy varieties.

The hot dog, long reviled by nutritionists, gained a measure of respectability once food scientists figured out how to transform soya-beans into a frankfurter. Veggie hot dogs, veggie burgers and veggie sausages debuted in health food stores but are now sold everywhere. Even deli meats have soya or wheat counterparts that look and taste very much like the real thing, with zero animal fat and cholesterol.

These foods are hardly the pinnacle of fine dining, but they are practical. If you have children, they are an absolute gift. If you saw what goes into a real hot dog, it would become the last thing you would want to see heading for your child's mouth. But a veggie version is something you can bring home with pride – and your kids will love them. These products help you through the transition to a broader range of healthy foods.

Soya milk has arrived big time. Once, buying soya milk meant shopping at a health food store that was dingy and dark. The cashier was wearing a tie-dyed shirt, his name was Sunshine, and folk music was playing in the background. Worst of all, the soya milk came in powder form, and you had to mix it with water and pour it on your cereal quickly before it precipitated.

Well, those days are gone. Health food stores are big businesses that know a thing or two about customer service. The folk music is gone, too, and there are a number of flavours of soya milk, along with rice milk, almond milk, oat milk and other varieties. Regular supermarkets stock these products, too, and people from all walks of life enjoy them.

As you shop for meat and dairy substitutes, take a look at the labels. When you check the ingredient lists, you will see that some products are not quite as vegetarian as you might like because they include egg whites or dairy proteins. Choose the vegan versions, and look for those that are lowest in fat.

COMPLETE NUTRITION

When you follow the nutrition guidelines in this chapter, your diet is likely to improve dramatically.[19] Not only will you skip all the animal fat and cholesterol, you will get much more of the healthy nutrients your body needs: soluble fibre to cut cholesterol, healthy vitamins to reduce cancer risk, potassium to lower blood pressure, and antioxidants to knock out free radicals, to name a few.

Even so, you are making a big change, and you are likely to wonder whether you are missing out on anything. Let me offer a word of reassurance. If you choose your meals from a variety of whole grains, pulses, vegetables and fruits and add any common daily multivitamin, you will have your bases covered.

Here's where the healthy nutrients are on your plate.

Protein. Your body uses protein to build and repair body tissues. Proteins are made up of small molecules called amino acids. All the proteins in your skin, muscles, bones and internal organs are built from various combinations of about 20 different amino acids.

A healthy diet of beans, grains, vegetables and fruits provides all the protein you need. In fact, you are better off getting protein from plant sources. While animal protein can be hard on the delicate tissues of the kidneys, plant proteins appear to be free of this problem. They are also free of the risks of calcium loss and kidney stones associated with animal protein.[20] Animal protein tends to cause calcium to pass through the kidneys and into the urine. In the process, calcium is not only lost, but it ends up in your urinary tract, where it can cause stones.

In years past, some nutritionists believed that vegetarians needed to carefully combine various foods in order to get adequate protein. The idea was that foods from plants might be missing one or more amino acids, so only combining foods in certain ways could ensure that you got them all. This notion was set aside long ago. The American Dietetic

Association's official position statements make it clear that plant-based diets provide plenty of protein without combining foods in any particular way.[21]

If, for any reason, you wish to increase your protein intake, turn to the bean group – you can find plenty of protein in soya products, such as tofu, tempeh and soya milk, and in wheat derivatives (e.g., seitan) used to make meat substitutes.

Calcium. For many people, calcium and milk are almost synonymous. They think that milk will build strong bones and protect against fractures later in life. Research has shown, however, that milk's benefits are, for the most part, a myth. The Nurses' Health Study, conducted by Harvard University, followed 72,337 women over an 18-year period to determine, among other things, whether milk drinkers had fewer hip fractures later in life. It turned out that those who drank the most milk had no protection whatsoever.[22] That's right. Women who drank three glasses of milk a day were just as likely to break a hip as women who never drank it.

How can that be? Well, only about one-third of milk's calcium is absorbed by the body. The other two-thirds simply passes out with the wastes. In addition, milk contains animal protein and sodium, both of which tend to increase calcium loss through the kidneys.

Do not misunderstand me here – you need some calcium in your diet, but it should come from healthy sources, namely green leafy vegetables and beans. While there is somewhat less calcium in broccoli than in milk, the absorption fraction – the percentage that your body can actually use – is higher for broccoli and nearly all other greens than for milk. There is one exception: spinach is high in calcium, but the absorption fraction is very low.

Greens and beans will give you the calcium your body needs. If you are looking for extra calcium for whatever reason, you can find plenty more in fortified juices and soya milks.

To maintain calcium balance, however, it is important not only to take in an adequate amount but also to minimize losses. Animal protein causes your body to lose calcium through the kidneys, and it can be measured in the urine. Studies of high-protein diets, such as the Atkins Diet, dramatically demonstrate the losses: such diets increased calcium loss by more than 50 per cent.[23] It is also important to limit sodium (salt) and get vitamin D from either sunlight or supplements. Vegetables and fruits promote bone strength for reasons that are not entirely clear, and exercise gives your bones a reason to live. It is a strong determiner of bone health. Finally, it is also important to avoid tobacco, since smoking increases fracture risk.

Iron. Iron is a double-edged sword. You need iron to build haemoglobin, which your red blood cells use to carry oxygen from your lungs to your body tissues. But too much iron can be toxic. It can increase the risk of heart problems and may even worsen insulin resistance.

Iron encourages the production of unstable molecules called free radicals, which can damage your body's delicate tissues and are linked to heart disease, cancer and even certain aspects of the ageing process.

The most healthy iron sources are the same foods that bring you calcium: beans and green leafy vegetables. They are rich in iron but carry it in a special form called non-haeme iron. Your body easily absorbs this form when it's in need of more iron, but the iron passes harmlessly out of the body when you have all you need. In contrast, meats contain haeme iron, which is like an uninvited guest at your party: it barges in whether you need it or not. Over the long run, meat eaters tend to accumulate too much iron.

If you are anaemic, do not rush out and buy iron supplements, or worse, add lots of meat to your diet. Instead, work with your doctor to find out what kind of anaemia you have and *why* it occurred. Anaemia can be a sign of kidney disease, it can be caused by certain drugs, and it can be a sign of blood loss from your digestive tract caused by gastro-intestinal irritation or even colon cancer. It is essential that you be evaluated and treated appropriately.

If you do need extra iron, turn first to greens and beans. Vitamin C–rich foods, such as fruits and vegetables, increase the absorption of iron from the other foods you eat, and avoiding dairy products helps, too. They are very low in iron and actually reduce its absorption from your digestive tract.

Zinc. Zinc plays important roles in immune function, wound healing and many other biological functions, but as with iron, you can have too much of a good thing. The most healthy sources include pulses, nuts and fortified breakfast cereals such as bran flakes.

Fat. Good fats, bad fats and too much fat – how do we make sense of it all? The most important fat fact is this: your body's actual fat requirement is minuscule, as you saw earlier. Most people in Western countries get many times the needed amount. With meats and dairy products front and centre in their diets, they not only get too much fat overall, they also get the wrong kind – *saturated* fat, which boosts cholesterol and aggravates insulin resistance.

Nuts, seeds, avocados, olives and full-fat soya products are also high in fat. Although they are low in saturated fat, the overall amount is high, and you should limit these foods accordingly.

As you also saw earlier, most vegetables, fruits and beans contain very little fat, and what they do have is a healthy mixture, including traces of the essential fats alpha-linolenic acid and linoleic acid.

If, for any medical reason, you are increasing your oil intake, healthy sources of omega-3 fats include walnuts, soya products, flaxseed and, in concentrated form, flax, linseed, rapeseed and walnut oils. Omega-6 oils are also sometimes used for health conditions such as arthritis, usually in the form of evening primrose oil, borage oil, black currant oil or hemp oil. They should be thought of as medicinal supplements rather than as foods.

Vitamin B$_{12}$. Your body uses vitamin B$_{12}$ to keep nerves and blood cells healthy. The amount you need is extremely small. The most convenient source is any typical multivitamin. You will also find it in many fortified breakfast cereals, fortified soya milk and other supplemented products.

Vitamin B$_{12}$ is not made by animals or plants but rather by bacteria and other single-celled organisms. How does this substance get from bacteria to the human body? We presume that before the advent of modern hygiene practices, there were traces of bacteria in the soil and on vegetables and fruits that provided tiny traces of vitamin B$_{12}$. In addition, bacteria in animals' intestinal tracts produce vitamin B$_{12}$, and traces of it end up in meat and other animal products. The problem with these sources is that along with it come cholesterol, fat and animal proteins. The sources listed above provide the B$_{12}$ you need without all that.

Vitamin D. Technically, vitamin D is not a vitamin at all. It's actually a hormone produced by sunlight on your skin, which is then converted to its active forms as it passes through your liver and kidneys. Once activated, it helps you absorb calcium and helps protect your cells against cancer, among other functions.

If you get plenty of sun, you do not need any vitamin D in your diet. Most of us are not that lucky, however. If you do not get regular sun exposure, taking a multivitamin containing 400 IU of vitamin D is important. Because of vitamin D's anticancer properties, some authorities call for higher intakes.

In the next chapter, you will get started with your new programme, and then, in Chapter 7, I will show you how to track your progress.

CHAPTER 5

How to Get Started

Take out a sheet of paper and jot down the headings 'Breakfast', 'Lunch', 'Dinner' and 'Snacks'. You are about to make a 1-day menu. Simply write down foods you like that meet the three guidelines set out in the previous chapter. In a nutshell, we are choosing foods that are:

Vegan: They contain no animal products. This means no meat, fish, dairy products or eggs – not even a little bit. The idea is to clean the animal fat, animal protein and cholesterol out of your diet. If you skipped to this chapter, please read the preceding one first. In this chapter, you will see how to make the shift surprisingly easy.

Low fat: You will use little or no added oil and omit other fatty ingredients. If you are reading labels, choose foods with no more than 2 to 3 grams of fat per serving.

Low glycaemic index: You will favour low-GI foods. This means generally avoiding sugar, white bread products, baking potatoes, most cold cereals and a few other foods. Most other vegan foods are fine. Certain foods have an especially low GI value: beans and other pulses, green leafy vegetables, most fruits, barley (which is great in soups) and the many foods that are made from them. Surprisingly, pasta has a low glycaemic index, unlike other wheat products.

HEALTHY BREAKFAST IDEAS

Under 'Breakfast', list breakfast foods you'd like to eat that are vegan, low in fat and low GI. Your list may well be similar to what you are eating already. Here are a few suggestions.

- Hot cereals such as oatmeal or wholegrain wheat cereal with cinnamon, raisins and/or apple purée or sauce (no milk)
- Cold cereals such as bran flakes with fat-free soya or rice milk and/or berries, peaches or bananas
- Melon, bananas or any other fruit
- Rye or pumpernickel toast topped with cinnamon (no butter or margarine)

If you like extra protein, try these.

- Veggie sausage
- Veggie bacon
- Scrambled tofu
- Breakfast tortilla wrap filled with 'refried' beans, lettuce and tomato (no egg or cheese)
- Baked beans or chickpeas
- Pumpernickel bread with hummus
- Any of the breakfast recipes beginning on page 191

Here are a few thoughts about some good breakfast choices.

Oats. Most of our research participants make old-fashioned porridge oats a part of their morning routine, and for good reason. Oats are rich in *soluble* fibre – the kind that gets creamy in water and removes cholesterol from your body. (Wheat and rice are high in *insoluble* fibre.) But that humble bowl of porridge does more than that. It helps bring your blood sugar under control and its high fibre content helps you lose weight.

An additional advantage comes from what oats *do not* have: cholesterol and animal fat. A bacon-and-eggs breakfast has a strikingly large amount of both.

Choose rolled or porridge oats, not instant or 'easy' varieties. Unlike quick-cooking types, old-fashioned oats have intact grains. The more intact the grain, the lower the GI, and the longer the cereal keeps you satisfied. See page 83 for tips on making the perfect bowl of hot oats.

For an extra blood sugar-lowering effect, top your bowl of porridge with cinnamon (see page 140 for details about how cinnamon affects blood sugar). Or add raisins, berries or just about any fruit or mix of fruits you like, but set the milk and sugar aside. Within just a day or two, you will break the habit of adding these unnecessary and unhealthy toppings.

If you just cannot imagine oats without milk, splash on some soya milk or rice milk; you will skip the animal fat and cholesterol of cow's milk.

Most dry cereals have a high GI, but oats are in the good GI range. They will keep you full and satisfied and help keep your blood sugar steady.

Veggie sausage or bacon. Ordinary sausage and bacon are loaded with cholesterol and fat and are among the most unhealthy foods on anyone's shopping list. But if you are unable to imagine breakfast without these meats, you are in luck. Food manufacturers have come to your rescue with vegetarian versions, and most supermarkets and all health food stores now stock them. If they are new to you, think of them as a liberal interpretation of the original; they are tasty and high in protein. Read the package labels, and choose those that omit animal ingredients (some are made with egg white, which is concentrated animal protein that you want to avoid) and are the lowest in fat.

Scrambled tofu. Tofu is almost identical to egg white – it has little flavour of its own but quickly takes on the flavours of whatever spices or sauces it is cooked with. Scrambled tofu is a great substitute for scrambled eggs – it has all the taste but no cholesterol, animal fat or animal protein. To add that all-important flavour simply add your favourite herbs or spices or see page 192 for a quick and easy recipe.

Breakfast tortilla wraps. No time for breakfast but you want something hearty? Wraps to the rescue. Simply grill them for a few seconds or pop them in the microwave, add beans, tofu, tomatoes or other favourite ingredients.

A Few Things Not on the Breakfast Menu

Just to state the obvious, eggs are off the list. A single egg has more than 200 milligrams of cholesterol – as much as an 8-ounce steak – plus a load of saturated fat, the kind that tends to raise cholesterol. The white of the egg presents a big dose of animal protein that you want to avoid. As you know, getting your protein from plant sources is better for your kidneys and your long-term bone health. Skip eggs and egg replacements that are made from egg whites.

Of course, breakfast meats are off the list, too, including 'lean' varieties. They *all* have cholesterol and animal protein.

Skip the bagel as well, unless you can find pumpernickel bagels. Yes, bagels are vegan and they are low in fat. But, similar to white bread, they have a high GI.

Forget doughnuts, Danishes and muffins. To see why, set one on a napkin for a few minutes, then look at how much grease has leached out. That grease is just waiting to fatten you up, boost your cholesterol and worsen your insulin resistance.

A Balanced Breakfast

You may wish to start your breakfast with a high-protein food such as veggie sausage and follow it with a starchier food like oats with cinnamon and raisins or a sweet food such as fruit. Here's why starting with a high-protein food can be helpful.

Starchy or sugary foods naturally increase the production of serotonin – the same feel-good chemical that is boosted by antidepressants such as fluoxetine (Prozac) and sertraline (Zoloft) – in the brain. Now, that's a nice benefit, but for some people, the result is post-breakfast drowsiness. In fact, some people actually use starchy foods as a remedy for insomnia. A high-protein food blocks the serotonin-producing action, boosting your energy. Any high-protein food will do: veggie sausage, veggie bacon, scrambled tofu, beans or even a spoonful or two of chickpeas – the kind you'd normally throw on a salad.

HEALTHY LUNCH IDEAS

Okay, let's move on to lunch. Here are a few ideas, but you will no doubt have many more.

Salads

- Green salad with fat-free dressing, lemon juice, or soy or teriyaki sauce
- Three-bean salad
- Pasta salad
- Kidney bean and sweetcorn salad
- Grain-based salad, such as noodles, couscous, bulgur or rice

Soups

- Asparagus
- Carrot and coriander

Sample 1-Day Menu

Breakfast

   Veggie sausage

   Rye toast

   Oats with cinnamon and raisins

   Sliced melon

Lunch

   Green salad

   Split-pea soup

   Hummus sandwich on rye bread with sliced tomato and cucumber

Dinner

   Spinach salad with cherry tomatoes

   Capellini (angel hair) pasta with tomato and mushroom sauce

   Steamed broccoli

Snacks

   Apples, oranges, bananas

- Minestrone
- Mixed vegetable
- Wild mushroom
- Lentil
- Vegetable chilli
- Split pea
- Spinach and nutmeg

Instant and prepared soups are okay as long as they are low-fat and free of animal products.

Sandwiches/Wraps

- CLT: sliced cucumber, lettuce and sliced tomato on rye bread with Dijon mustard

- Hummus on a wholemeal pitta with grated carrots, beansprouts and sliced cucumber

- Sandwich made with low-fat meat alternatives such as veggie turkey, chicken or ham slices, plus your favourite sandwich veggies on rye bread

- Spicy salsa dip, canned cannellini or kidney beans, red pepper and tomato slices and lettuce wrapped in a wholewheat tortilla

- Italian aubergine sub: baked aubergine slices, pizza sauce and 'sautéed' mushrooms on a wholegrain sub roll

- Any of the lunch recipes beginning on page 212

Extras

- Fresh fruit
- Chickpeas
- Cut-up vegetables

Here's a rundown of good lunch choices.

Salads. Salads vary from the simple lettuce-and-tomato variety to pasta salads, three-bean salads, fruit salads and many others.

If you start with salad greens, everyday lettuce such as cos or little gem is fine, but do not shy away from fresh spinach, watercress, rocket and other greens. Add cucumber and tomato slices and by all means, chickpeas, kidney beans or other pulses to your salad. They provide plenty of nutrition and are great at holding your blood sugar steady.

For convenience, supermarkets stock three-bean salads in tins, which are ready when you are. Many stores also have well-stocked salad bars.

When you choose dressings, look for fat-free vegan varieties, which you should be able to find at many supermarkets.

Soups. Soup is a great lunch starter, or a big bowl of hearty soup can *be* your lunch. Loaded with vegetables, beans, barley or other grains, and wonderful flavours, soups are satisfying and wonderfully healthy. If you cook up a big pot on the weekend, you will be ready for the week ahead.

If you are looking for convenience, dried soup mixes are timesavers – but check the label to ensure they're vegan. If you like, add tomatoes or any frozen or fresh vegetables. Stir a tablespoon or two of nutritional yeast into each bowl for a savoury touch. If you add extra carrots, tomatoes, frozen vegetables (e.g., broccoli, kale, cauliflower or green beans) and spices, you will turn your soup into a stew.

If you'd like to let someone else do the cooking, your supermarket has an endless variety of tinned and fresh soups. You need to be selective, but you will find plenty that meet our requirements. Lentil, minestrone and vegetarian vegetable are good choices.

To have homemade soup anywhere, pick up an insulated bottle, such as a Thermos, so you can just fill it with soup and take it to work. Your colleagues will wish they had done the same.

One caveat about prepared soups: some manufacturers overdo it with salt, so it pays to choose lower-sodium brands. Aim to keep your total daily sodium intake to less than 2,000 milligrams.

Sandwiches. Sandwiches are quick and portable, and with the enormous variety of ingredients available these days, they can be healthy, too.

Start with a lower-GI bread, such as rye or pumpernickel. Try any or all of the following fillings.

Hummus is a Middle Eastern dish that has become hugely popular. Unfortunately, many commercial brands are too high in fat, but who needs them? With a food processor, it takes only about 5 minutes to make your own, and a big batch will last for days. See page 200 for recipes.

Vegetarian cold 'meat' slices mimic the taste of chicken or ham with none of the animal fat or cholesterol. They are sold at all health food stores and many supermarkets, and they make great sandwiches. You can find them next to the vegetarian sausages, which are also great choices. As always, choose lower-fat brands.

Veggie burgers are easy to make, and commercial brands are widely sold in health food stores and supermarkets. Be aware, however, that the content of veggie burgers varies widely and some are high fat and contain egg as a binding agent – so check the label.

A BLT made with veggie bacon, lettuce, tomato and mustard is a great choice. My own keep-it-simple sandwich is a CLT, made on toasted rye bread with lettuce, sliced cucumber and tomato, sometimes a slice or two of vegan 'meat', and topped with mustard.

Speaking of condiments, mustard is fat-free; make it your spread of choice. Most mayonnaise spreads are just the opposite – they are loaded with fat. You can buy very low-fat mayonnaise but it is not vegan so should also be avoided.

Frozen meals. While there are endless rows of standard ready meals available, vegan frozen meals are still mainly the preserve of small specialist producers who sell their products on the internet, though you should be able to find a limited number in your health food store.

If lunch means dining out – or perhaps fast food – see Chapter 8 for healthy choices.

HEALTHY DINNER IDEAS

There is a limitless array of healthy foods for dinner, whether you like to cook or not. Many people enjoy cooking, but many others feel too busy or just cannot be bothered; they tend to choose simple and convenient foods or eat out. Personally, I fall squarely into the second group, while Bryanna Clark Grogan, who developed the recipes for this book, is just the opposite. She is so skilled in the kitchen that it looks like fun, not work.

The good news is that both kinds of people do very well in this programme. Here are a few ideas for starters.

- Classic tomato pasta: some commercial tomato sauces are fine. Choose those lowest in fat and free of animal products. Favour whole wheat pasta. Add some broccoli or spinach (prepared fresh or frozen), and you will be set

- Beans and rice: try kidney beans mixed with salsa and cooked rice and sprinkled with coriander. Black beans are also a good choice and are becoming much more widely available

- Soft tacos: start with a wholewheat tortilla and add beans, lettuce, tomato and salsa

- Veggie lasagne: use low-fat tofu to replace the cheese and add layers of grilled veggies

- Ratatouille risotto: mix tinned ratatouille through cooked rice and add artichoke hearts, asparagus tips and mushrooms

- Oriental stir-fry: use a nonstick pan to fry tofu and vegetables and season with low-sodium soy sauce

- Low-fat vegetarian burgers: read the labels and choose those lowest in fat and free of cheese and other animal products

- Fajitas: lightly sauté sliced peppers, onion and aubergine in a nonstick pan and add a little garlic and a pinch of cumin and chilli powder.

- Stew made with chunky vegetables in a savoury sauce

- Mushroom stroganoff

- Any of the wonderful and easy-to-prepare dinner recipes beginning on page 223

There is no need to be nervous if you are not a cook – there are plenty of convenience foods and restaurant meals that will fit the bill. Our job for now is not to make you into a chef, but simply to make a realistic 1-day menu of foods you really will eat and enjoy.

Ethnic foods are often great choices, whether you make them yourself or have them at restaurants: Mexican bean burritos, Italian pastas and bean soups, Chinese vegetable and rice dishes, Japanese vegetable sushi with miso soup and salads, Indian curries, Thai dishes and many others. These foods take advantage of the fact that plant-based diets are much more common in other countries than they are in Europe and North America.

If your idea of dinner is sending out for pizza, it can still be vegan and low in fat. Just ask for all-vegetable toppings, such as mushrooms, peppers, onions, sun-dried tomatoes and capers. Avoid the cheese and ask for extra tomato sauce instead. If you are making pizza at home, you can add veggie 'meat' slices if you like.

SIMPLE SNACK IDEAS

Okay, your day's menu is nearly complete. But even if you feel you will not be hungry between meals, pencil in a few snack ideas so you will be ready in case the munchies do hit. A 3:00 p.m. hunger pang can erode your resolve, so stock up on things that you can feel good about eating. Here are some snack suggestions.

Fruits have a surprisingly low GI in most cases, and they are unbeatable for nutritional value. Keep apples, oranges, pears, bananas and other fruits on hand. Some people like to keep a bowl of melon chunks in the refrigerator for an instant snack that's ready when they get home. Dried fruits are acceptable. Surprisingly, their GIs are not necessarily higher than those of fresh fruit. Because their water has been removed, however, it is easy to take in far more calories with dried fruit than with fresh fruit, so it pays to favour the fresh varieties.

Instant soups are great to keep in your desk drawer; just add hot water when you are ready to eat. Minestrone, split pea, lentil and other varieties are typically vegan and low in fat.

A simple sandwich of lettuce and sliced cucumber and tomato with mustard on rye bread will fill you up, with nothing to regret.

Three-bean salad will hold you until dinner.

Air-popped popcorn skips the fat of the usual kind. Try sprinkling it with nutritional yeast.

Hummus on a wholemeal pitta is filling and low in fat if you use the quick recipe on page 200.

Other simple snacks include bran cereal with soya milk, pumpernickel or rye toast with jam, carrot sticks and rice cakes.

CHOOSING YOUR MENU FOR THE COMING WEEK

All right, you are doing great! You have made good choices that will give you a healthy start. Let's look ahead at the next week. Pencil in some breakfasts, lunches, dinners and snacks for the next 7 days. It is fine to repeat items, use leftovers or make your life easy in any way you can. Remember, though, do not limit calories or skip meals.

It is essential to be realistic. If you do not enjoy cooking now, that is unlikely to change. Plan to have foods on hand that require little preparation.

A Balanced Dinner

A good way to make sure your dinner is well balanced is to fill about a quarter of your plate with a pulse dish. That means beans, peas or lentils. You might choose baked beans, chickpeas or cannellini beans for example. These foods are rich in protein, soluble fibre and minerals and have wonderfully low GIs.

Next, fill another quarter of your plate with a starchy food such as brown rice, sweet potato or pasta. *Starch* is an unglamorous word, but it really means complex carbohydrate – the healthy, clean-burning fuel that powers your body.

Finally, fill the remaining half of your plate with vegetables. Ideally, choose two different varieties – say, a green vegetable like broccoli and an orange vegetable like carrots. These foods are your nutrition powerhouses. Add fruit for dessert and you will be set.

You can vary these proportions if you like. As long as your plate is vegan and low in fat and has a low GI, you will be fine.

There are a million ways to do this. Some people like an Italian or Mediterranean meal, which might include bean soup and pasta with a chunky vegetable sauce. Some favour an Oriental dinner, with tofu (which counts as a pulse because it is made from soyabeans), rice and vegetables. An Indian-inspired plate might include a lentil curry with rice and vegetables.

When I visit my parents, we substitute a bean dish and vegetable cutlets for the usual meat dish and add sweet potatoes and vegetables. Dessert might be pears, strawberries or oranges. See the pattern? It's still there: a bean dish, a starchy food for healthy carbs, vegetables and fruit for dessert.

Will you be at work? Travelling? Planning ahead is essential. If there is nothing healthy in the company canteen, you will want to pack a lunch. Sometimes when a colleague asks what I am having for lunch, I answer, '*les restes d'hier*'. This sounds exotic until I explain that the phrase is actually French for 'leftovers'. But the fact is, my leftovers sometimes *are* exotic, depending on which restaurant filled the doggie bag!

Let's Go Shopping

Okay, now that you have your menu, it is time to go shopping. Your goal is to stock your shelves with the foods and ingredients you will need so your week goes smoothly. And when hunger hits, you will be ready.

Take a trip down those aisles at the supermarket that you may well have neglected in the past. The produce department may stock meat substitutes, soya milk and other healthy products, along with an ever-growing array of new and interesting fruits and vegetables. Also check out the 'health' and 'free from' aisles. And look at the shelves with innumerable varieties of rice and colourful dried beans.

Be sure to check out your nearest health food store if you have not done so already. You will find substitutes for meat, cheese and milk and interesting foods from other countries, all worth a try. Explore and experiment; some new finds will become favourites. If the occasional purchase turns out to be a dud, do not worry. That is what experiment-ing is all about.

As you shop, pick up ingredients that will allow you to prepare a few extra things at the weekend – a pot of soup or stew, for example – that you can then split into portions for quick reheating during the week.

You will notice that prices for healthy foods vary widely. Overall, vegetarian foods are less expensive than meaty or cheesy products. Beans, fresh and frozen vegetables, pasta, rice – these humble ingre-dients cost very little. However, health food stores sometimes put premium prices on prepared products, which is true for non-vegetarian as well as healthy vegan items. You will soon sort out your best choices.

While you are at the health food store, pick up a daily multivita-min. As you have seen, it's important to get adequate vitamin B_{12} and a multivitamin is a great way to do that. The best ones are iron free and vegetarian.

SOME STAPLES: BASIC FOODS TO TASTE AND TRY

There are a few basic foods that would be good for you to get to know. They are not elaborate – just simple, basic staples that ought to be on your shelves. If they are new to you, they will be healthy additions to your repertoire. Let me list some here and encourage you to think about them when shopping.

Old-fashioned oats. Choose porridge oats over instant and see how easy and fast they are to prepare. Just combine 1 part oats with 2 parts cold water, bring to the boil and simmer for a couple of minutes. That's all there is to it. Oats are loaded with soluble fibre to bring your cholesterol down and filling enough to keep hunger at bay all morning. While you are at the supermarket, pick up some toppings: cinnamon, raisins or other fruit – grated apple or pear is particularly good.

Beans. Get to know the many varieties of this humble food. Very low in fat; devoid of cholesterol; high in soluble fibre, calcium and iron; and with an enviable glycaemic index, beans' day has arrived. Cook them up from scratch if you like, but it's handy to stock your shelves with the wide array of tinned beans now available – cannellini, haricot, flageolet, black, kidney, borlotti, black-eye and any other varieties you see.

Frozen vegetables. *Convenience* is the word here. If you are the slightest bit pressed for time, you will be glad you have vegetables in your freezer that just need a little steaming. Nutritionally, frozen vegetables are equivalent to fresh. Look for broccoli, spinach, brussels sprouts, carrots, cauliflower and anything else you fancy.

Lentil soup. Lentils assert themselves in a hearty and healthy soup. Keep a tin or two on hand.

Hummus. This simple chickpea dip has become an enormously popular sandwich filling. But skip the commercial brands, which are too high in fat (even the reduced-fat varieties). If you have a food processor, you can make your own in less than 5 minutes, and you will be set for the week. Check the recipe on page 200 and pick up the ingredients the next time you go shopping.

Chickpeas. Speaking of chickpeas, this is one pulse that is really at home just about anywhere – not just as hummus but also in salads, soups, pasta sauces and stir-fries. You can even eat them for breakfast. Keep a few tins on your shelf.

Toppings. Dijon mustard is great for sandwiches and lemon juice or cider vinegar are great on green vegetables and salads. Salsa was just made for beans, and fat-free dressings of any variety are handy, too.

Brown rice. Many people have never tasted a properly prepared bowl of rice. The trick is to select brown rice, toast it slightly, and cook it like pasta, using what may seem like too much water and draining away the excess at the end.

Barley. This grain is all over the breakfast cereal aisle, in puffed and sugared form, but barley really shines in soups and stews or when served as a grain side dish. You can mix it with rice and cook them together. Barley has a low GI, lots of soluble fibre and wonderful taste and texture.

Tomato sauces for pasta. Take a few minutes to read labels on jars of plain tomato sauce to find varieties that exclude animal products and keep oil to a minimum. Then stock your shelves for a quick and easy dinner. Pick up your favourite pasta to go with it.

Meat substitutes. Try the veggie versions of hot dogs, burgers and 'meat' slices. They are not haute cuisine, but they serve a useful purpose and some taste surprisingly similar to the foods they imitate. Read the labels, though, and skip products with animal-derived ingredients or more than 2 to 3 grams of fat per serving. Health food stores usually have the best selection, but many regular supermarkets stock some, too.

Nutritional yeast. You can find this in the supplement aisle at health food stores. Nutritional yeast dissolves into pasta sauces, stir-fries, casseroles, soups and lots of other recipes, adding a subtle cheese-like taste. It is not the same as brewer's yeast or baker's yeast, both of which taste bitter. Nutritional yeast comes in flakes and powder. For better texture and versatility, buy the flakes.

Fresh fruit. Fresh fruit is a perfect snack, and you will want to keep it on hand, but you cannot keep it for long. Be realistic and choose what you are likely to eat.

What to Do with Unhealthy Foods?

So you have filled your shelves and refrigerator with healthy staples. If some not-so-healthy items from your previous diet are still lurking, though, what do you do? That's easy: get rid of them. Give them away, throw them away or feed them to your cat. But do not keep tempting foods nearby. They present more of a temptation than you need.

Planning Ahead

Eventually, healthy eating will become second nature. For now, though, you will need to put a bit of thought into where you will be at lunchtime and dinnertime and what you will have. There really are healthy choices out there, but they are sometimes not so obvious in a culture that caters to unhealthy tastes. It helps to plan ahead.

ON YOUR MARK, GET SET . . .

As discussed in the last chapter, you will want to pick out a 3-week period and really dive into this new menu. Choose a time when you have the mental energy to embrace a change. If you are an accountant, the end of the tax year probably is not a good time. If you are a student, exam week may not be the best choice. But once you have picked your time, jump in with both feet. Do the diet change 100 per cent. Follow our three guidelines as closely as humanly possible, and do it all the way.

Check the Label

There are two things you want to look for on product labels. First, check the ingredient list to make sure there are no animal-derived ingredients. Common ones include milk solids, whey, casein (and various casein derivatives, such as sodium caseinate), egg products and gelatine. Also be on the lookout for partially hydrogenated vegetable oils, which are as bad as saturated fat, and are found in many processed goods.

Sometimes people want to make exceptions for foods that *sound* as if they are healthy. Honey, for example, has gotten unjustified good press over the decades. Nutritionally speaking, honey is simply sugar, offering you nothing from a health standpoint. Rather like olive oil, its marketing has gotten way ahead of its value.

Next, check the Nutrition Facts. Ideally, a serving of a food will have no more than about 2 grams of fat.

If label reading seems a bit cumbersome, keep in mind that you need to check a product only once. As you find the products that fit the bill, there's no need to check them again. Also, simple foods do not need labels. No one ever had to look for the fine print on a banana or pear, a bag of frozen spinach or a bag of frozen broad beans. Each of these foods has exactly one ingredient.

Okay, you have done great. You have the basics down. In the next several chapters, we will look at specific health issues and situations you may encounter, and I will offer plenty of tips for handling them.

CHAPTER 6

Healthy Weight Control

If you have been aiming to lose weight, let me show you the steps that make the process as easy, effective and permanent as possible. For anyone – but especially for people with diabetes – eliminating unwanted weight is tremendously important. For starters, it boosts your insulin sensitivity; the more body fat you trim away, the more responsive your cells are to insulin. This is especially true for fat around your waistline.

Weight loss also brings down your cholesterol and blood pressure. And when you've trimmed away body fat, exercise is that much easier and more inviting. Your joints – especially your knees – will thank you.

Needless to say, there are a great many ways to lose weight. In the US, many diabetics follow the American Diabetes Association (ADA) diet guidelines. These work for some people, but others find the approach a real challenge because it relies on calorie limits. If you normally eat 2,000 calories per day, for example, the ADA recommendations would limit you to 1,500 – and that gets tiresome very fast. If you're hungry at 8 in the evening and you've already had your 1,500 calories for the day, you will go to bed hungry. That will never happen on the programme recommended in this book.

Low-carbohydrate diets are potential disasters for anyone, but especially for people with diabetes. They often bring short-term weight loss, but most of the weight quickly returns. Low-carb diets also have wildly unpredictable health effects. In research studies, as many as one-third of low-carb dieters have shown a significant increase in LDL ('bad') cholesterol. Some have had such high cholesterol levels that they have been forced to drop out of studies.

What's more, low-carb diets are usually high in protein. The animal protein that is commonly emphasized in these diets can be hard on your kidneys. Harvard researchers tracked kidney function in 1,624 women participating in the Nurses' Health Study, focusing especially on those who had any loss of kidney function at the start of the study. It turned out that the more animal protein the women consumed, the more kidney function they lost.[1] Given that about 40 per cent of people with diabetes have already lost some kidney function, it makes good sense to protect yourself from further damage.[2] I strongly caution against any diets that recommend high-protein foods.

As you have seen, such diets are based on the outdated idea that avoiding carbohydrates is the key to glucose control. As you know by now, populations that make rice, noodles and other carbohydrate-rich foods their diet staples actually have had very little obesity and very little diabetes. Low-carb diets can cause weight loss over the short run, but there are far healthier ways to achieve that goal and to make weight loss last over the long run.

A healthy approach to weight loss focuses on choosing the right kinds of foods, not on the *quantity* of food you eat. When you have the right foods on your side, the calories and portions fall into line on their own, and weight loss is almost automatic.

A WEIGHT-LOSS DIET THAT WORKS

In 2005, my research team published the results of an important study that tested a new and powerful approach to weight loss. The partici-

Say No to Low-Carb Diets

Weight loss lowers cholesterol levels. On average, each half a kilogram or pound you lose lowers your cholesterol level about 0.3 mmol/l,[3] so most weight-loss diets improve your cholesterol test results. The exception is low-carbohydrate diets. They are so high in fat and cholesterol that they increase cholesterol levels for about one in every three dieters, some of whom have eventually experienced wildly high cholesterol levels and serious heart disease symptoms.[4,5] There is no good reason to begin any low-carbohydrate, high-protein diet.

pants were women with moderate to severe weight problems. Most had tried many different diets: low-calorie diets, low-carb diets, Weight Watchers, the cabbage-soup diet and just about everything else. Like most people, they had found these diets difficult to follow, and whatever weight they lost soon returned.

Our approach was very different. It did not include calorie counting, limits on portions or carbohydrates, or even an exercise prescription. For research purposes, we wanted to isolate the effects of diet.

The participants lost weight easily, averaging about 0.5 kg (1 lb) per week – week after week after week.[6] When we used a similar diet in people with diabetes, we found much the same thing. In a 12-week study, the average participant lost 7.2 kg (16 lb).[7]

So how does it work?

First of all, it is important to understand where the calories are hiding in the foods you eat. A chicken stores extra calories in chicken fat. A cow stores calories in beef fat. A fish stores them in fish fat. Body fat – in humans or animals – is a calorie-storage system.

If you were to remove a bit of fat from a drumstick or chicken wing and send it to a laboratory, you would find that a gram of fat – that's $\frac{1}{28}$ ounce – has 9 calories. That is a lot. It is more than double the calories in a gram of carbohydrate – the starch in rice, beans or sweet potatoes, for example. Carbohydrates have only 4 calories per gram. Small wonder that people who make rice or other plant foods their staples tend to stay slim. Throughout Asia and rural Africa, rice and other grains, root vegetables and various pulses are the traditional foundation of the diet. These foods are filling but have relatively few calories.

Of course, it's a different story in Europe and North America, where meals feature meat and dairy products, which contain the very fat that animals have used to store their excess calories. Weight problems are the all-too-common result. If you want to avoid taking in extra calories, you would do well to avoid eating the concentrated calories that animals have hidden away in their body fat.

Thus, step one is to avoid animal products. If you do that, you will of course avoid animal fat completely.

Step two is to keep vegetable oils to a minimum. Beans, grains, vegetables, fruits and most other foods from plants have very little fat. There are a few exceptions, however: nuts, seeds, olives, avocados and some soya products are high in fat. Keep them to a minimum as well.

Be especially careful about vegetable oils. Now, some people argue that plant oils are more healthy than animal fats, and it's true that they are much lower in *saturated* fat, the kind that raises cholesterol levels and is linked to breast cancer and insulin resistance. When it comes to weight problems, however, animal fats and vegetable oils are essentially all the same. They all pack in 9 calories per gram.

Step three is to focus on high-fibre foods. A grain of brown rice, for example, has a thin cloak of fibre surrounding the grain that gives the rice its tan colour. To produce white rice, manufacturers strip away this coating, but you are better off if it is left intact. Fibre, which was once called roughage, fills you up so you feel naturally satisfied after a meal.

As you saw in Chapter 4, each 14 grams of fibre added to your daily menu cuts calorie intake by about 10 per cent on average.[8] That simply means that high-fibre foods fill you up faster, so you stop eating sooner. Instead of trying by sheer force of willpower to cut calories, you cut them *without even thinking about it*.

The richest sources of fibre are beans, vegetables, fruits and whole grains. While breakfast cereal commercials tend to push grains as the best fibre source, you will find much more fibre in beans and most vegetables than in most grains. But they all add up. Aim for at least 40 grams per day. One caveat: if high-fibre foods, especially beans, have not been part of your routine, try gradually upping the amount you eat to give your digestive tract time to adjust. See Chapter 9 for more tips on avoiding digestive problems.

In the next chapter, I will show you an easy way to check your fibre intake using the Quick Fibre Check.

Okay, let's summarize: to lose weight, you want to avoid animal products, limit the use of vegetable oils and go high fibre. Vegetables, fruits, whole grains and beans fit the bill perfectly.

HEALTHY EXAMPLES

By now, you already have a good idea of what this looks like on your plate, because the diet changes for weight loss are very much like those for diabetes. Breakfast might start with veggie sausage or veggie bacon – that is, faux meats made of soya or wheat – followed by a big bowl of oats or perhaps some fresh fruit. You would skip bacon, eggs and muffins and bagels, which are stripped of fibre.

Steps to Weight Loss

1. Avoid animal products. If you steer clear of fish, chicken, beef, dairy foods and all other animal products, you will cut your animal fat intake to zero. What's more, this shift will mean that you will naturally eat high-fibre foods to replace those from animal sources, which have no fibre.

2. Keep vegetable oils to a minimum. If you have a bottle of cooking oil in your kitchen, throw it away. There are simpler and better ways to cook (see page 185). Also limit nuts, seeds, olives, avocados and full-fat soya products.

3. Favour high-fibre foods. Build your meals around beans and other pulses, vegetables, fruits and whole grains.

To ensure complete nutrition, take a standard multivitamin each day.

Lunch could be a sandwich made with sliced tomato, lettuce and hummus on rye. A pasta salad would be fine, too.

For dinner, you might try tomato or split-pea soup followed by a vegetable stir-fry or vegetarian shepherd's pie filled with chunky vegetables. In the process, you will avoid animal fat, have very little vegetable oil and get all the fibre in those healthy vegetables.

For a between-meal snack, an apple or banana fits the bill nicely, while potato crisps or nuts pack too much fat. You will find plenty of fresh ideas in the Menus and Recipes section.

Vance

When Vance joined our study, he wanted to get his weight down to 95–102 kg (15–16 st). Since he initially weighed in at 125 kg (19½ st), he had a long way to go. He stuck to the diet programme, however, not worrying about calories or portions but paying close attention to the types of food he chose. Everything was vegan and low in fat. Also, in order to give the diet a good test, he agreed not to add any exercise for the first 6 months.

The weight started to come off. Three months later, he weighed in at 114 kg (17 st 9 lb) – a loss of 11.3 kg (1 st 8 lb) in about 12 weeks. Friends couldn't help but notice and many asked him what his secret was. After 6 months, he was down to 108 kg (17 st). At the 14-month mark, he was at 98 kg (15½ st).

Nancy

Nancy began the study at 89 kg (14 st). Like Vance, she changed her diet but kept her activity level the same to allow us to test what the diet change alone could do. Three months into the programme, her weight was down by 6.4 kg (1 st). After 6 months, she had lost 11.3 kg (1 st 8 lb), and at 14 months, she weighed 70.3 kg (11 st) – a loss of nearly 19 kg (3 st) without counting calories.

FOODS THAT WORK MAGIC

These simple foods have surprising effects. Not only do they help you trim hundreds of calories off your daily menu, they also cause a fundamental change within the cells of your body. As you saw in Chapter 2, clinical tests have shown that they increase your body's after-meal calorie burn. The reason is this: as you change your diet, your insulin

Not Exactly Health Food

A few years ago, I was running a study on diet and weight loss and found that a couple of our participants were snacking on Twizzlers – a red sweet that comes in long twists like licorice. When I asked why they were eating sweets, they pointed out that the product is both vegan and low in fat. And sure enough, there's a friendly message printed on a package of Twizzlers Strawberry Twists:

> Did you know . . .
> Strawberry Twists are a low-fat candy! That's right, the same great-tasting Twizzlers you have known and loved are low in fat, as always. Nothing has changed.

A look at the ingredients list shows that indeed, nothing *has* changed. The corn syrup, flour, sugar, cornstarch, partially hydrogenated soyabean oil, salt and artificial flavour are all still there. Like other sweets, it is basically a sugary concoction containing nothing that your body even remotely needs. Without any fibre to fill you up, foods like this can really pack in the calories.

If you find Twizzlers or other sugary sweets on your shelf, it helps to remember the third guideline in this programme. We choose foods that are not only vegan and low in fat but also low GI. Sugar is nowhere near as high in calories as fat, but it still provides more calories than you need.

sensitivity begins to improve. That means that glucose has an easier time entering your cells to be burned for energy, rather than continuing to circulate in your blood.[9] The after-meal calorie burn is small, but it lasts for about 3 hours after each meal, giving you an extra edge for losing weight.

USING VOLUMETRICS

Barbara Rolls, PhD, a researcher at Pennsylvania State University, has proposed an innovative way of thinking about appetite control called Volumetrics.[10] Her studies have looked at what triggers satiety – the sense of fullness after meals – and shown how to plan meals to bring on a feeling of satiety earlier.

Surprisingly, what makes us stop eating does not seem to be the number of calories we have ingested, nor is it the number of grams of carbohydrate or protein in a meal. Rather, it is the *weight* of food we have taken in. It is as if your stomach has a scale, and once it registers a certain number of grams of food, it signals your brain that you have had enough.

We all tend to eat roughly the same weight of food each day. If your meals do not add up as they normally do, your appetite guides you to have a little more.

There's an effective weight-loss strategy in there. If the foods you eat contain a fair amount of water – soups or fruit, for example – they are heavy enough to tip your 'stomach scale' and reduce your appetite. Because the weight of these foods comes mainly from water, which has no calories, they tend to cut your total calorie intake for the day.

Dr Rolls uses the term *energy density* to describe how many calories are packed into a food. A food that has a lot of water has a low energy density. That is, it has very few calories per kilogram or pound.

If it helps to favour foods that hold water, what would be some good choices? Here are a few.

- **Soups.** These are filling but generally low in calories. Favour clear, low-sodium soups rather than creamy varieties.

- **Salads.** Add tomatoes, chickpeas, cucumbers, peppers and other vegetables to make a salad into a meal while keeping it low in calories. Use fat-free dressing, lemon juice or cider vinegar rather than regular oily dressings.

- **Fruits.** Apples, oranges and pears are heavy compared to other foods and have few calories.

- **Vegetables.** Vegetables of virtually any variety are good choices. Adding chunky vegetables to salads and casseroles increases their volumetric power.

- **Bean dishes.** Think of chilli and casseroles.

- **Whole grains.** Rice beats rice cakes. Pasta beats bread. In each case, one is water based and filling, while the other is airy and not filling at all.

Including these foods generously in your menu will accelerate your weight loss.

One important caveat: for some reason, simply drinking water will not turn off your appetite. Your stomach apparently reacts differently to heavy foods – which trigger an appetite shutoff – than to a drink of water, which does not.

Dr Rolls proved this with an interesting experiment. She invited volunteers to eat a bit of casserole as an appetizer and then measured how much lunch they ate afterwards. In her experiment, the volunteers consumed an average of about 400 calories at lunch. If they ate the casserole appetizer along with a glass of water, they again ate about 400 calories at lunch. In other words, adding the glass of water did not change anything. In a third test, however, she stirred the glassful of water into the casserole to make soup. When she measured the participants' calorie intake afterwards, she found it was cut to less than 300. The soup tricked their stomachs into shutting off their appetites.

While foods that contain water as a major ingredient are good, there are other foods that are not so good. You will want to steer clear of those that are rich in either fat or air. Fatty foods such as meat, cheese, potato crisps and onion rings are filling, but they pack a lot of calories. As you recall, fats have 9 calories in each gram.

Airy foods – such as melba toast, pretzels and bread – are not especially high in calories, but they will not fill you up, either. You can eat serving after serving of these foods without feeling full. The idea is to have a food that is low in calories *and* filling.

Good Volumetric Choices

Here are some tips for reducing the energy density of your meals.

- Choose fresh fruit or old-fashioned oats for breakfast.

- Add chunky vegetables to salads and use fat-free dressing, lemon juice or vinegar.

- For soups, choose stock-based (not cream-based) varieties.

- For snacks or dessert, enjoy fresh rather than dried fruit. Remember that fruit is better than crackers or pretzels.

- Add chunks of courgette, squash, peppers, onions, or aubergine to sauces or pizza.

There's an easy way to check the energy density of commercial food products: just take a look at the label. If one serving has fewer calories than grams, it is a good choice. For example, the label on a tin of black beans (below) shows that a serving has 90 calories and weighs 122 grams, so the beans are a good choice. They are a volumetric food.

Black Beans

Nutrition Facts

Serving Size: 122 g

Servings Per Container: Approx 3½

Amount Per Serving:

Calories 90 Calories from Fat 5

An 80 gram serving of spinach has just 17 calories, so it's also a winner. Each of these foods has less than 1 calorie per gram, so the weight of the food fills you up before the calories fill you out.

What about skinless chicken breast? One serving has 173 calories and weighs about 100 grams (3.5 ounces). Not a good choice. Aside from not being vegan or particularly low in fat (23 per cent of calories), it has far more calories than grams.

A slice of bread may have 80 calories and weigh 32 grams. It has few calories but is very lightweight, so it is not filling. With more calories than grams, it is not especially helpful for weight loss.

I am not suggesting that you use Volumetrics in place of the other diet guidelines in this book. Use it in addition to this programme to ramp up the weight-loss power of your new menu. Volumetrics will help you pick from among the allowed foods those that are the most filling with the fewest calories.

Again, the idea is simply to reduce the *energy density* of the foods you eat by choosing those that naturally contain a fair amount of water to fill you up and shut off your appetite.

WHAT TO EXPECT

Everyone loses weight at his or her own pace. In our studies using low-fat vegan diets, weight loss averages about 0.5 kg (1 lb) per week. In turn, each half kilogram or pound you lose tends to reduce your cholesterol level by an average of about 0.3 mmol/l.[11] Adding exercise can increase the pace, depending on your regime.

You may find that you lose weight, then reach a plateau and stay there for a while. If that happens, see if there is something in your diet you can change, such as eliminating hidden sources of oil or boosting your fibre intake. Our bodies seem to have different plateaus depending on the fat content of our foods. That is to say, if you drop the fat content slightly, your weight will probably drop a bit, then plateau. If you drop the fat content more, you'll drop down to a new plateau.

The same thing works with fibre. Do a Quick Fibre Check (page 107), and if you're not up to 40 grams per day, try adding more beans, vegetables, fruits and whole grains to your diet. You'll find that the combination of steering clear of fats and bringing in fibre helps trim away the weight.

Take Your Time

If you have gradually gained weight over the years, let it come off gradually. Don't starve yourself in the hope of instant results. If you are on an optimal diet and are physically active, nature will take its course. As the weeks go by, you will not only be slimmer, you will also be healthier. Your cholesterol and blood pressure are likely to fall along with your blood glucose. As always, stay in close touch with your doctor so your medication doses can be revised as you regain your health.

CHAPTER 7

How to Track Your Progress

In this chapter, we will look at the various tests that allow you to track your progress. The first one, glucose testing, is particularly important, but please read through the whole chapter. It will help you stay on track. We will start with blood tests and then look at other kinds of testing, including weight, blood pressure and examinations of the eyes and feet.

GLUCOSE TESTING

Monitoring your blood sugar is essential to controlling diabetes. Glucose is measured in milligrams per decilitre (mg/dl) in the United States and in millimoles per litre (mmol/l) in most of the rest of the world.

If you have type 1 diabetes or are using insulin for type 2 or gestational diabetes, you should check your glucose at least three times a day or according to whatever schedule your doctor recommends. If you have type 2 diabetes and are using oral medications, there is no optimal testing frequency. As a rule of thumb, however, when your diet, medications, exercise routine or health status changes, it is important to test more frequently. If your doctor is not yet aware that you are about to make a change, now is the time to share that information. You should also discuss what to do if your blood glucose is too high or too low. As you begin a healthy diet, your numbers are likely to fall significantly.

Regular glucose testing is especially important if you are taking diabetes medications, particularly insulin or medications that cause your body to release insulin. The reason is that these are powerful drugs that actively push your blood sugar down. And you are now starting a powerful new diet. The combination of these treatments – drugs *and* diet (sometimes along with exercise) – may end up pushing your blood sugar too low.

I know what you may be thinking: impossible! If all you have ever heard from your doctor is that your blood sugar is too high, it's hard to imagine it could fall too low. Well, it can. *The combination of a powerful diet and the diabetes medications you may already be on can be very strong.* In fact, your blood glucose can fall so low that you start to shake and sweat (see below for other symptoms). This is called hypoglycaemia. In rare cases, people who make a major diet change or embrace a strenuous exercise programme without backing off on medications find their blood sugar drops dangerously low – so low that they can lose consciousness. This is why it is essential that your doctor be made aware of the changes you are making – so your medication dosages can be altered if your blood glucose takes a nosedive.

Dangerous hypoglycaemia is very unlikely if you are on no medications, and it is also unlikely if you are being treated with only metformin (Glucophage) or a thiazolidinedione, such as rosiglitazone (Avandia). However, hypoglycaemia is *likely* to occur if you take any of the following drugs.

- Insulin (any injected, pump or inhaled form)

- Glipizide (Glibenese, Minodiab)

- Glimepiride (Amaryl)

- Nateglinide (Starlix)

- Repaglinide (Novonorm)

This is just a short list of medications that may put you at risk. Ask your doctor if the medications you are taking may cause hypoglycaemia.

Although hypoglycaemia is a sign that your body is regaining its insulin sensitivity – which is of course a good thing – it is also a sign that your medicines are now too strong and that you need to speak with your doctor right away about adjusting your medication regime. If your doctor has stopped your medications, hypoglycaemia is very unlikely to occur.

Symptoms of hypoglycaemia include:

- Shaking

- Sweating

- Hunger

- Anxiety

- Weakness

- Rapid heartbeat

- Dizziness or lightheadedness

- Sleepiness or confusion

- Difficulty speaking

If you experience these symptoms, check your blood sugar. If it is below 3.9 mmol/l or whatever other benchmark value your doctor recommends, you need to eat something that raises your blood sugar quickly. If you notice symptoms while driving, pull over to a safe spot. And if you are unable to test your blood sugar or are unsure whether it is low, assume that it is low and have something to eat. Glucose tablets are a great choice. They are sold at all pharmacists, and you will want to keep them in your bag or briefcase and in your glove compartment. If your blood sugar check shows you are hypoglycaemic, you should take 15 grams of glucose. If you have typical glucose tablets with 4 grams of glucose each, you will need to take four tablets at once. Here are some other good choices.

- 120 ml (4 fl oz) of any fruit juice

- 120 ml (4 fl oz) of a regular (not diet) soft drink

- 5 or 6 pieces of hard confectionery such as fruit drops

- 1 or 2 teaspoons of sugar

After 15 minutes, check your glucose again. If it is still below 3.9 mmol/l, have another serving, then check again in another 15 minutes. If you are within an hour of mealtime, go ahead and eat. If not, have a snack. Be sure to carry glucose tablets or a quick-energy food with you

Carl's Hypoglycaemic Episode

Carl had been taking metformin and glipizide for about 5 years, and his morning blood glucose values ranged between 6.7 and 8.3 mmol/l. He changed his diet with the hope of coming off his medications, and in fact, very soon after he began this programme, his readings began to drop. After about 2 weeks, they were often under 5.6 mmol/l. Carl was delighted with such clear evidence that the changes were working.

About a month into the diet, he had an unusual experience. One morning at about 10:00 a.m., he found himself feeling unusually hungry. He always had a good appetite, but this was something different. He felt ravenous. Over the next several minutes, he started to tremble and broke into a sweat. 'Oh, yes,' he thought to himself. 'This is what they told me might happen.' He checked his blood glucose, and it was 3.6 mmol/l, which is lower than it should be. He had some orange juice and an early lunch. He telephoned his doctor, who reduced his glipizide dosage. Over the next several weeks, the episodes repeated several times. Eventually, his doctor stopped the glipizide altogether.

Carl's morning blood glucose readings stabilized at around 4.4 to 5.0 mmol/l. He never needed to go back on glipizide, and he never had another hypoglycaemic episode.

for emergencies, wear a medical identification bracelet, and be especially attentive to your glucose level during exercise, which can cause blood sugar to drop.

Hypoglycaemia can also occur while you are asleep. Look for these signs.

- Nightmares or crying out
- Finding that your pyjamas or sheets are damp from perspiration
- Awakening with unusual tiredness, confusion or irritability

If these occur, you can check for night-time hypoglycaemia. Simply set your alarm for about 2:00 or 3:00 a.m. and check your blood sugar a few nights in a row. Consult your doctor to see if you need a medication change.

Hypoglycaemia does not mean there is anything wrong with your diet. Rather, it means that the medication regime you are on has become too strong for you. The next step is to contact your doctor, who will probably reduce your medication dosages or eliminate one or more drugs. Get in touch with your doctor as soon as you can – if possible the same day the episode occurs. Do not put it off, because the hypoglycaemic episodes are likely to recur until your medications are reduced.

To track your blood sugar, use a logbook or a simple grid like the one below.

Blood Glucose						
DATE	MEDICATION REGIME	EARLY	BREAKFAST	LUNCH	DINNER	LATE
			/	/	/	
			/	/	/	
			/	/	/	
			/	/	/	
			/	/	/	
			/	/	/	
			/	/	/	
			/	/	/	
			/	/	/	
			/	/	/	
			/	/	/	
			/	/	/	
			/	/	/	
			/	/	/	
			/	/	/	
			/	/	/	
			/	/	/	
Note: It is especially helpful to check your blood glucose before meals. Mark these numbers to the left of the slash marks. Mark after-meal values to the right of the slash marks.						

Making Sense of Glucose

Blood glucose values are a bit like the stock market: although they generally follow a trend, they can bounce around from day to day. Certain situations can trigger an unexpected rise. Any sort of illness or infection can boost your blood glucose; even a minor upper respiratory illness or a scraped foot can cause a significant jump in your numbers. Stress can too, due to the action of stress-related hormones.

Having some up-and-down swings in blood sugar is normal, but if your glucose remains high day after day, it will lead to high HbA1c, which increases the risk of complications. The American Diabetes Association recommends that people with diabetes use the following guidelines for blood glucose levels.

- Fasting or before meals: 5.0 to 7.2 mmol/l
- One to 2 hours after a meal: 10.0 mmol/l
- At bedtime: 5.6 to 7.8 mmol/l

The Dawn Phenomenon and the Somogyi Effect

You may occasionally be surprised to find that your blood glucose is higher in the morning than it was when you went to bed the night before. Or perhaps you checked your glucose in the early morning and then went back to sleep, only to find that it had risen while you slept. How is this possible?

No, sugarplums dancing in your head had nothing to do with it. The fact is, your body constantly monitors and alters how much glucose is in your bloodstream. Glucose is vital to your body's functioning – especially to the workings of your brain – so your body has a way of increasing your blood glucose when it gets a bit low. In the early-morning hours – typically between 5:00 and 9:00 a.m. – hormones (growth hormone, cortisol and catecholamines) cause your liver to release glucose into the bloodstream. These hormones can also interfere with insulin's efforts to remove glucose from the blood. This 'dawn phenomenon' can noticeably raise your blood sugar.[1]

A similar reaction can occur when a person using long-acting insulin has an unusual blood glucose dip in the middle of the night. Let's say, for example, that you miss your usual late-night snack and the insulin you are taking forces your glucose level too low. Once again, your natural hormones will compensate, raising your blood sugar. This is called the Somogyi effect. It is different from the dawn phenomenon in that it is triggered by an overly low blood sugar level occurring in the middle of the night.

Although your body has a system for controlling your blood sugar, it is a bit imprecise. Your blood sugar can still run too low or too high despite your body's best efforts, and you will occasionally see a high or low level that you cannot explain.

HbA1c BLOOD TEST

As discussed in Chapter 1, the main test for assessing your progress is an HbA1c blood test. Your HbA1c level should be checked every 6 months, or every 3 months if your diet, medications, or general health are changing or if previous values have been too high. If your HbA1c is high, your doctor will be concerned, and you should be, too. If it is low, you are doing well. To give you a frame of reference, Diabetes UK says that HbA1c should be less than 7 per cent and, for individual patients for whom further reductions are possible, closer to 6 per cent. Many people regularly attending diabetes clinics in UK health centres manage to achieve the 7 per cent goal: it is harder to keep consistently under 6 per cent, but it is worth trying.

A typical oral diabetes medication brings HbA1c down by an average of about 1 point or a bit less. The effect of a good diet on HbA1c varies depending on how good your control is when you start, how well you follow the diet and how much excess weight you lose. Your result will also be affected by exercise, genetics and other factors.

The biggest drops we have seen in short-term research studies are on the order of 3 or 4 points in approximately 6 months. These are seen in people whose HbA1cs were high (say, 9 or 10) to begin with. People whose HbA1cs are in the 7 to 8 range are likely to have a drop averaging between 1 and 2 points. People who continue to lose weight beyond this time could have an even greater drop, assuming they were not already in the normal range.

The higher your HbA1c, the greater your risk of circulatory problems. Evidence suggests that keeping HbA1c low is particularly important for the health of your eyes and kidneys and for preventing nerve symptoms.

From your heart's standpoint, a 1-point increase on the HbA1c scale – from 7 to 8 or 8 to 9, for example – brings about a 20 per cent increase in your risk of heart problems over about a decade.[2] In other words, if you had a 10 per cent risk of having a heart attack sometime in the next decade, a 1-point rise in your HbA1c, maintained over the whole decade, would boost your risk to 12 per cent. A 2-point rise would mean a 14 per cent risk and so on. What these numbers tell us is that HbA1c is important and that by all means, you will want to aim to get your HbA1c down. However, HbA1c is not the sole key to good health. To stop diabetes from attacking your heart and blood vessels, you will also want to focus on your blood pressure, cholesterol and weight. Needless to say, your doctor can and should track these values with you.

FRUCTOSAMINE

Fructosamine is an intermediate-term measure of blood glucose control. Whereas HbA1c reflects your control over the preceding 8 to 12 weeks, fructosamine reflects your control over the preceding 3 weeks or so. Doctors use it much less often than glucose or HbA1c. In the UK, it is not done routinely, except in research or in exceptional circumstances in special clinics.

CHOLESTEROL

Your doctor will check your cholesterol at regular intervals, at least once a year. As you will see in Chapter 12, high levels of cholesterol in the blood can damage your heart, major blood vessels and the delicate blood vessels of the eyes and kidneys. Here are the numbers to aim for.[3]

Total cholesterol. In the US, the government's National Cholesterol Education Program states that total cholesterol should be below 5.2 mmol/l. I suggest you aim for a considerably lower goal, however. In large population studies, it is clear that the lower your cholesterol, the lower your risk of heart problems, until you reach a threshold of about 3.9 mmol/l. In the UK, six of the biggest organizations who deal with cardiovascular disease have recently formulated new guidelines (the Joint British Societies' guidelines) that state that people with diabetes should aim for a cholesterol level of less that 4 mmol/l. My suggestion is to use 3.9 mmol/l as your goal.

Low-density lipoprotein (LDL) cholesterol. LDL cholesterol is often called bad cholesterol because it raises your risk of heart problems and other blood vessel complications. According to the Joint British Societies' guidelines, your LDL cholesterol should not be higher than 2 mmol/l if you have diabetes, however some scientists are pushing for even stricter standards below 1.8 mmol/l for high-risk patients. Some authorities in the US have called for lowering your LDL by 30 to 40 per cent regardless of what your starting level is.[4] Your risk of heart problems drops as LDL decreases, until you reach a level of approximately 1.0 mmol/l.[5]

High-density lipoprotein (HDL) cholesterol. HDL cholesterol is often called good cholesterol because it carries cholesterol out of the body. Generally speaking, the higher your HDL cholesterol, the better. Current goals are to have an HDL level above 1.2 mmol/l for men and above 1.4 mmol/l for women.

Some doctors, however, interpret HDL in the context of your total cholesterol concentration: in this case, a favourable HDL reading would be at least one-third of your total cholesterol. For example, if your total cholesterol is 3.8, a healthy HDL would be 1.3 or above. This is an important consideration because many people who follow healthy diets do not have much of *any* kind of cholesterol – LDL, HDL, or anything else.

Triglycerides. Triglycerides are tiny fat particles transported in the bloodstream. Normal triglyceride concentration is less than 1.7 mmol/l.

See Chapter 12 for information on controlling cholesterol and triglycerides.

CHECKING YOUR KIDNEY HEALTH

Because your kidneys can easily be affected by diabetes, your doctor will check your kidney health with a simple urine test at least once a year. The goal is to see whether your kidneys are losing protein, specifically a protein molecule called albumin. Albumin itself is not especially important. What is important is that if it shows up in your urine, it is a sign that your kidneys have been affected by diabetes and are not holding on to albumin as they should. Albumin losses of greater than 30 milligrams over 24 hours are considered abnormal. Your doctor will also check your blood for creatinine and estimate your glomerular filtration rate and will interpret the results of these tests for you. For more on factors that influence kidney health, see Chapter 13.

OTHER ROUTINE LABORATORY TESTS

Your doctor will run other tests to track your progress. The following are two very common ones.

Full blood count (FBC). This test shows the state of your blood cells. Many people with diabetes develop anaemia, meaning they have fewer red blood cells than they should. A full blood count lets your doctor easily check this and many other measures. If your blood count is low, your doctor will investigate the reasons for it, which could include kidney disease, iron deficiency, use of certain medications, abnormal bleeding or other factors.

Biochemistry profile. A routine biochemistry profile is also known by several other names. It assesses your overall health, with a special focus on the status of your kidneys and liver, and lets doctors check for potential adverse effects from medications.

There is no reason to despair if any of your laboratory values are not where they should be, but it is definitely a reason to take action. You will want to optimize your diet and work with your doctor to plot a course for tracking the effectiveness of your overall health regime.

TAKING STOCK OF YOUR DIET

I would like to shift gears now and look at your diet and overall health. First, let's take a minute to make sure that your diet is going according to plan.

• Are your foods vegan? You know you are doing well if there are no foods of animal origin on your plate, not even little bits of fish, skimmed milk or egg white – nothing. If you have done this right, there is *no* animal fat, *no* cholesterol and *no* animal protein in your diet. Your menu is built around plant foods and it is rich in fibre and all the healthy nutrients the plant kingdom brings you. If you need a refresher on why you are doing this, please take another look at Chapter 4.

- Are your meals all low in fat? It is important to really keep fats and oils to an absolute minimum. Be careful with nuts and nut products.

- Are your foods low GI? The main problem foods are sugar, corn syrup (a sweetener used in some processed foods), white and whole-meal breads (favour rye and pumpernickel) and baking potatoes (choose sweet potatoes and yams).

Quick Fibre Check

One way to help gauge how you are doing is with the Quick Fibre Check. It is a handy little tool and I suggest that you do one about once a week as you begin this new approach to eating. Scoring is simple and takes only a minute or two to learn. Soon, estimating the fibre content of virtually everything in the supermarket will be easy. You will also see if you are getting enough fibre in your daily menu. It does not take long, and it will help you see if you are on track.

First, take a minute to jot down everything you ate or drank for one full day on the form below. I will explain below how to fill in the fibre column.

Food (one food or ingredient per line)   **Fibre**

_____	_____
_____	_____
_____	_____
_____	_____
_____	_____
_____	_____
_____	_____
_____	_____
_____	_____
_____	_____
_____	_____
_____	_____
_____	_____
_____	_____
_____	_____
_____	_____
Total	_____

Then, next to each food, note its fibre score, using the following guide.

Beans: For each serving of beans or lentils (one serving = 115 g/4 oz) or any food that includes about this amount of beans or lentils as an ingredient, give yourself a 7. A 240 ml/8 fl oz serving of soya milk or 90 g/3 oz of tofu (both made from soyabeans) rates a 3.

Vegetables: For each serving of vegetables (one serving = approximately 140 g/5 oz or a good handful), give yourself a 4. An exception is lettuce, for which the same amount scores a 2. A potato with skin scores a 4; without the skin, a 2.

Fruit: For each medium piece of fruit (e.g., an apple, orange or banana; a banana smoothie), mark a 3. For 240 ml/8 fl oz of juice, mark a 1.

Grains: For each piece of white bread, bagel or equivalent, score a 1. Wholemeal breads score a 2, as does 140 g/5 oz of cooked pasta. A 170 g/6 oz serving of rice scores a 1 for white and a 3 for brown. 125 g/4½ oz of cooked oats scores a 4. Score a 3 for typical ready-to-eat cereals, a 1 for highly processed cereals, and an 8 for bran.

Interpreting Your Score

Total your fibre score and let's see how you are doing.

Less than 20: You need more fibre in your diet. As it is, your appetite will be hard to control and you may have occasional constipation. Boosting fibre will help tame your appetite and cut your risk of many health problems.

20–39: You are doing better than most people in Western countries, but as you bring more fibre into your diet, you will find that it makes foods more satisfying and cuts your calorie intake a bit.

40 or more: Congratulations! You have plenty of healthy fibre in your diet to control your appetite and help keep you healthy. Fibre also reduces your risk of developing cancer, heart disease, diabetes and digestive problems.

CHECKING YOUR WEIGHT

Of all the things that predict success in dealing with diabetes, leaving behind excess weight is among the most important. The strategy outlined in Chapter 6 is a highly effective way to go about it. Here are some tips for tracking your progress.

- First, track your weight. Some people who have been overweight for a long time have not gone near a set of scales in years. If that sounds like you, give it another try. It is essential to know if you are losing weight. If not, it is time to change course. Usually, that means tuning up your diet. Weight loss is sometimes difficult, and genetic tendencies do play a role, but your diet is one thing you really can control.

- Use the same scales each time you weigh yourself. Different scales can give dramatically different readings.

- Check your weight at the same time of day each time. With food and water intake, you can easily gain and lose a little weight in the course of a day. Usually, you will be heavier in the evening.

- In gauging the success of your weight loss, about half a kilogram or 1 pound per week is a healthy goal. It is about what you can expect if you follow the diet presented in this book without doing particularly vigorous exercise. Slower weight loss is also fine as long as you are moving in the right direction.

- Do not rely on exercise alone for weight loss. A healthy diet change can easily trim 300 to 400 calories a day off your daily menu, but burning that many calories through exercise means walking or running *3 or 4 miles a day*. Exercise is important, but it cannot begin to take the place of diet changes.

TRACKING YOUR BLOOD PRESSURE

Maintaining healthy blood pressure is extremely important. As you can imagine, increased pressure inside your arteries can damage the arteries themselves, as well as your heart, eyes, kidneys and nerves. The longer your blood pressure stays high, the more damage it can do.

Problems can travel in the other direction, too: damage to the kidneys can lead to high blood pressure. The reason is that your kidneys play an important role in regulating your blood pressure, and if they have been assaulted by diabetes, they can lose some of their ability to do this.

In Chapter 12, we will look at how diet affects blood pressure. For now, here are your targets.

Normal blood pressure is defined as 120/80 millimetres of mercury (mm Hg) or less. The current UK guidelines ask doctors to try to maintain blood pressure in diabetes at less than 120/80 mm Hg. This will often mean taking more than one type of blood pressure-lowering drug. The aim is to protect the kidneys from the effects of high blood pressure, and if there are signs of kidney involvement (albumin in the urine and/or an eGFR below 60) then this target blood pressure is especially important.

Have your blood pressure checked regularly. If it is not where it should be, take another look at your diet and speak with your doctor about what, if any, additional treatments you may need.

CHECKING YOUR EYES

You should have your eyes checked for signs of diabetes in your retina ('retinopathy') and your lenses (cataracts) once every year. In Britain, ophthalmic optometrists are highly trained to do this, and will pick up the signs more effectively than your doctor can. As a person with diabetes you should already be on the priority list for annual eye examinations. They will normally be done by your ophthalmic optometrist (the new name for an optician) who will refer you to your doctor if your eyes show any signs of diabetes-linked deterioration. Once you are known to have diabetic eye complications, your hospital diabetes eye specialist unit will follow you up, too.

If you smoke, tell your eye doctor. Yes, you will get a lecture, and it is time to listen up if you are still smoking. See Chapter 13 for information on the effects of nutrition on eye health.

CHECKING YOUR FEET

Foot problems are common in diabetes. If your blood glucose has been poorly controlled, you are at risk of developing neuropathy – nerve damage – which means you may not be aware of small injuries to your feet. Wound healing may be slowed as well. Small injuries can gradually worsen and become infected.

For this reason, you not only want to get your diet into shape by following the guidelines in this book, you also want to have your doctor check your feet at least once a year. The examination will include a check for sensation using a thin plastic thread, a check of your vibratory sense with a tuning fork, and a thorough check for any signs of damage to your skin. Take the advice of Mary Ellen Wolfe, RN, a nurse working with George Washington University, who recommends that you take off your shoes and socks at every doctor's visit to be sure your doctor does not forget to examine your feet.

STAYING HEALTHY

No matter how healthy you get, you should still keep an eye on your glucose, HbA1c and cholesterol; weight; eyes; and feet. But I hope that as you tune up your diet and lifestyle, that is all you will be doing – just confirming that all is just as it should be.

CHAPTER 8

A Perfect Diet in an Imperfect World

It is not always easy to follow a perfect diet in an imperfect world. There will be times when those you depend on – restaurants, airlines, colleagues and even family members – have little understanding of or interest in healthy foods. This chapter is dedicated to these situations. I will cover dining out, travel, social situations, working with your doctor and dealing with family members. When life puts obstacles in your way, I will show you how to tackle them with ease.

DINING OUT

Dining out is part of life and you ought to be able to enjoy a night on the town with friends or loved ones without missing a beat on your new healthy diet. Luckily, many restaurant menus offer plenty of healthy selections. Unfortunately, others are limited. Often the key to success lies in where you go as well as what you order when you get there. Here are a few tips.

First, think international. In Mediterranean countries, Asia and Africa the traditional dietary staples are grains, vegetables, pulses and fruits. Not surprisingly, all of these regions have historically had much lower rates of diabetes than Western Europe. When you choose from the best of what these cuisines have to offer, dinner out can be both healthy and delicious.

Italian restaurants are everywhere, and they would love to serve you spaghetti marinara, minestrone, pasta e fagiole (a traditional pasta and bean soup), healthy salads, chunky vegetable and tomato pizza, grilled broccoli and steamed spinach. Because their foods are often made to order, it is easy for chefs to minimize oil, leave off cheese and so on.

Chinese restaurants will get you started with vegetable spring rolls or vegetable pot sticker dumplings and various healthy soups. Favour the steamed, not fried, items. Skip the meat dishes and get right to the long list of savoury vegetable main dishes made with tofu (also known as bean curd), green beans, broccoli, spinach and other healthy ingredients. The danger in Chinese restaurants, as in most eating establishments, is overexuberance with the use of oil. Ask that your food be prepared with as little oil as possible and have your main dish along with plenty of rice, preferably brown rice.

Japanese restaurants are among the very best choices when it comes to healthy dining. Sushi chefs are delighted to transform carrots, cucumbers, radishes and other simple ingredients into edible delights. Have them along with miso soup, salads, seaweed and various appetizers.

Thai and **Vietnamese** restaurants serve many vegetable dishes that include rice, soft noodles, vegetables and tofu along with wonderful sauces.

Indian restaurants are mixed. While vegetarian diets are traditional and highly respected among many Indians, the use of oil and dairy products often puts them in the no-go zone. Your best choices are soups, rice dishes and vegetable curries prepared with minimal oil.

Ethiopian restaurants are not common but if you are lucky enough to get the chance to dine in one don't miss it. Because some religious groups in Ethiopia follow vegan diets during certain times of the year, the restaurants serve many dishes made with chickpeas, split peas, lentils, green beans, peppers and delightful spices. They will be happy to serve you all their vegan items on a large platter for a wonderful dinner.

Steakhouses and gastropubs are obviously trickier places to find vegan food, however most have salad bars or salad on the menu and offer plenty of vegetables. Pasta can also be a good option.

Second, ask for what you want. If what you are looking for is not on the menu, do not be afraid to ask. Most restaurateurs will gladly alter their main offerings to accommodate a special request. If you would like cheese and bacon bits left off your salad, if you would like a vegetable selection, or if you would like your pasta topped with tomato sauce instead of meat sauce, by all means, ask. You will not only get a better meal, you will also help the restaurant management understand how to better serve patrons like you.

As I noted above, restaurant kitchens often overdo it with oils, so ask your waiter how foods are prepared and request that your meal be made with as little oil as possible. In Italian restaurants, spinach and broccoli are often sautéed, but they can also be steamed. The same goes for most Asian vegetable dishes.

Sauces and condiments can always be served on the side. This goes for pasta sauces, salad dressings, brown sauces used in Asian cuisine, spreads used on sandwiches, and similar items.

Ask for what you want. You will be glad you did.

Fast Food

Fast food is rarely a top choice when the priority is healthy eating. On the other hand, these chains are big businesses that understand the growing demand for healthy food choices. More and more often, you do find offerings on their menus that will fit into a healthy diet. Burger King, for example, offers a veggie burger that is much lower in fat than its other sandwiches. Another good choice is the Veggie Delite at Subway.

Some fast-food restaurants offer salad bars. With chickpeas, three-bean salad, cherry tomatoes and chopped vegetables, a salad becomes a hearty meal.

In that vein, one of the best ways to get healthy food fast is to stop at any large supermarket and patronize its salad bar. A wealth of great choices is right at your fingertips.

Nancy's and Vance's Experiences

Nancy often dined with friends who liked good food and good restaurants. I encouraged her to choose ethnic cuisine – Chinese, Japanese, Italian or Thai, for example. Unfortunately, that was not what most of her friends had in mind, and they felt uncomfortable knowing she would not eat unhealthy things.

When she headed out to join friends at a restaurant that might not be very accommodating, she often had a snack in advance so she would not be starving when she got there. When she went to friends' houses for a meal, she often volunteered to take a vegetable dish and some fruit salad.

On a holiday to Iceland, she packed granola bars and individual soya milk cartons in her luggage, just in case she needed them as occasional meal supplements. She got by just fine.

'I am tempted sometimes, especially when I am stressed or overtired. I talk myself out of it,' she said.

She found it helpful to keep things in perspective. 'You have to decide what your priorities are,' she explained. 'I didn't want to suffer from the effects of the disease. I wanted to stop the progression. I didn't even think about reversing it. And now I'm a walking advertisement for the programme. People keep asking me how I've done it. I've described it in detail to probably 40 people.'

When Vance dined out, he looked for veggie burgers, fresh steamed vegetables and pasta without cheese and oils. His challenge was sports stadiums. 'I love going to baseball and football games, where french fries, hot dogs and soft drinks are about all that's offered. It would be great to be able to take in healthy food or even just some carrot sticks and a bottle of water, but usually they don't allow any food to be taken in. So at first I stuck to pretzels and popcorn. At one game I smelled the fish and fries, and it was hard to resist,' he said.

Veggie hot dogs and burgers came to Vance's rescue. Although they are not necessarily the ultimate dining experience, they are a major improvement on the foods they replace.

TRAVEL

Travel presents challenges no matter what kind of diet you follow. Here are a few ways to help keep your new eating plan on track.

Choosing restaurants wisely. As you have seen, there are usually plenty of vegan choices at non-vegan restaurants, particularly those that feature international cuisine. Even some fast-food places can rise to the occasion.

You might go online to check out vegan and vegetarian restaurants in cities you are planning to visit – if they have a website rather than just a restaurant listing you may even be able to check the menu in advance. There's no reason to limit yourself to these restaurants, though; almost any eating establishment should be able to accommodate you.

Before you fly. When you are booking a long flight (or generally up to 48 hours before your flight), request a vegan meal. You will get a healthy meal and will often be served first.

On many short flights, meal service has gone by the wayside, so you might pick up some easy-to-pack snacks at a health food store or supermarket. Vegetarian 'meat' slices are great sandwich fillers and resist spoiling. Individual cartons of soya milk or rice milk need no refrigeration. A pack of hummus with pitta bread, a few pieces of fresh fruit, some baby carrots, instant soup (flight attendants will gladly provide hot water), or a small tub of chickpeas can be lifesavers.

SOCIAL EVENTS

It can be tough to stick to the plan at parties, even when you know you will regret a slip in the morning. If you arrive at a party unprepared, there may well be nothing available that you can eat. With a bit of planning, though, you can celebrate without leaving the healthy path you are on. Here are some ideas.

Offer to take a healthy dish. Let's say you have been asked to a friend's home for dinner, and you have no idea what they will serve. Here is what I suggest: when you get the invitation or as soon thereafter as possible, call your hosts to let them know that you have changed your diet and that you do not want to put them to any trouble. Say that you would like to bring something, such as a low-fat hummus dip or an exotic fruit salad. I can almost guarantee that your hosts will say there is no need to worry and you need not bring anything because there will be plenty to eat. Now, regardless of what they were really thinking, you have alerted them to your needs without imposing in the slightest.

If you are reluctant to let your hosts know, do not be. They will be much more embarrassed if they find out after the fact that they served a dinner with nothing you wanted to eat. Besides, you are very likely to find that other guests — and even your hosts — are making similar diet changes.

Take a healthy gift. Instead of the usual bottle of wine, why not arrive with a healthy food gift? A fruit basket, a loaf of artisan pumpernickel bread or a healthy party dip will delight your hosts and ensure that you have something to eat.

Avoid arriving hungry. If you arrive ravenous, you will be drawn to the unhealthy foods. If you eat something before you arrive, you will be fine.

Carry a plate. At buffets or drinks parties, guests with nothing in their hands are inviting others to offer them something. Make yourself a plate with a few crudités or a bit of bread, and no one will be inclined to offer you foods you do not want to eat.

AT THE DOCTOR'S OFFICE

Medical care is a partnership; you and your doctor need to work together to best meet your needs. This is true at any time, but especially when you are in the process of changing your diet. The fact is, your diabetes will probably be improving, and you will need to keep a close watch on your medications.

Some doctors are not easy to reach, and even if you have your doctor's attention, that does not mean he or she wants to engage in a conversation about nutrition. Some doctors show little interest in the topic, while others have frankly outdated or untested ideas about it.

I suggest you lend a copy of this book to your doctor with a sticky note flagging Chapter 14. It was written for doctors and shows them the scientific rationale for the diet presented in this book, the evidence behind it, and what they can anticipate.

You can help by holding up your end of the partnership. That means following your doctor's advice (provided it is sound and you agree with it), letting him know how you are doing, calling him promptly if your blood glucose drops below 3.9 mmol/l or whatever other criterion he sets, and taking a multivitamin so he will not worry about you developing any sort of deficiency. The truth is, your nutrition is much better on a vegan diet than on an omnivorous diet, but a knowledgeable doctor will want to be sure you are getting your B_{12}. A multivitamin will easily take care of that.

In the vast majority of cases, doctors are absolutely delighted when their patients improve their diets. They are all the more delighted when they see the improvements on the scales and in laboratory results.

One of our research volunteers thought his doctor would be sceptical about his plans. They talked about little aside from blood tests and prescriptions during his appointments. To his surprise, however, when the doctor found out he was starting a vegan diet, she was delighted. 'That will probably help you a great deal,' she said. And indeed, it did. Within 6 months, he lost 13.5 kg (2 st), he was able to stop one of his two diabetes medications and he was continuing to improve week by week. His doctor had no formal education in nutrition, but she knew success when she saw it. She now recommends the same diet to other diabetes patients.

LOVED ONES WHO HELP AND HURT

Sometimes our friends and family members help us stay on a healthy path. When we are not enthusiastic about exercising, they encourage us by going with us. When we are tempted by some less-than-healthy food, they shore up our resolve.

Improving our diets is like quitting smoking or breaking any other habit – we need our family's support. But sometimes, intentionally or unintentionally, our loved ones are not so helpful. They may not be aware of the risks of a bad diet, or perhaps they are all too aware and are struggling with unhealthy habits of their own. They may even try to sabotage your efforts to break bad habits.

If the problem is that your loved ones simply do not have much information about healthy diets, lend them this book. If they are not eager readers, try this little trick: put a sticky note or bookmark at any page you think they would find of special interest. They will be drawn to that section, and once they start reading, they will probably continue.

If family members tease you about your eating habits, remind them how important your health is to you. Explain that it is tough for you to have unhealthy foods around and that you really need their help. Ideally, they will join you in your new, healthy way of eating. If they just will not change, then at a minimum, they must keep their food separate and not tease or tempt you with unhealthy items.

GOOD FOOD FOR THE WHOLE FAMILY

If you are preparing meals for your family and they are balking at new foods, do not despair. It is natural to be cautious about anything new. Present healthy foods without pushing them and recognize that it often takes a couple of tries before a new item really catches on.

I suggest that you not fix healthy meals for yourself and less-than-healthy meals for your spouse or children. Some people do this, figuring they cannot change others' bad habits. But remember this: not only will introducing healthy foods to your family bring you some very important allies, it will benefit your loved ones as well as you.

The very best situation is when the whole family decides to change together. There is no health reason for anyone to eat animal-derived foods, fatty foods or sugary foods. Yes, these foods are everywhere in modern societies, but they are the principal reason for the epidemics of overweight, heart disease, cancer and other health problems in Western nations. When the whole family makes the same diet change, they all get the same advantage.

One good way to break through resistance is to ask your family members to try a short-term diet change with you as an experiment. Say that you'd like to try new and healthy ways of eating for just 3 weeks, and you would like them to join you. Most people will try anything for a short period. By the time 3 weeks have passed, they will have sorted out the new foods they like and will be ready for more.

When introducing healthy foods to children, it is generally best to stick to simple, familiar items. Some children may not yet care for exotic vegetables, but they will easily gravitate to sweetcorn, carrots and peas. Avoid wrangling with a child who is reluctant to try a new food. Sometimes altering the form of the food makes a huge difference. A child who does not care for the texture of cooked spinach may like fresh spinach as part of a salad. Steamed broccoli and cauliflower may be intimidating, but they may be perfectly acceptable when chopped and added to a soup or stew. Kids may not go for lentil loaf, but they love veggie burgers and hot dogs and sandwiches made with vegetarian 'meat' slices.

It always helps to present choices. Would your children prefer baked beans or lentil soup? Would they prefer their veggie burgers cut into halves or quarters? The idea is to give kids a sense of control while all the possibilities are good ones.

In some families, food is a symbol of affection. Parents stuff their children with sweets and gooey desserts, as if love could be measured in calories. Whatever the motivation, none of this does you one bit of good. Find other ways to express affection. A book, a walk, a trip to the movies – there is no shortage of meaningful gifts.

HEALTHY FOODS IN AN UNHEALTHY WORLD

A visitor from another planet might well conclude that modern civilization has no perceptible interest in healthy diets. Fast-food restaurants – and many other restaurants – carry lots of fatty, cholesterol-laden meals and far fewer healthy choices. Television commercials push endless less-than-healthy snacks. Convenience stores and snack machines offer lots of what you do not want and precious little of what you do want. Sometimes, you may feel like a person who is trying to quit smoking but is trapped in a bar where cigarettes are free.

In large part, you would be right, but truly, there are also plenty of healthy options. For every convenience store selling unhealthy food, there is a supermarket with an ever-expanding range of great food products. For every restaurant that refuses to serve anything health-conscious eaters would look for, there are a dozen that offer good choices. The range of health-oriented cookbooks is truly enormous, and it is now easier than ever to follow a healthy diet. Friends and family members – even those who do not follow healthy diets themselves – all know that what you are doing is worth supporting.

CHAPTER 9

Troubleshooting

How are you doing with your new way of eating? Are you reaching your weight-loss goals? Are your glucose and HbA1c coming down? Is your cholesterol improving?

If you are having any sort of trouble, this chapter will guide you through the most common problem spots.

NOT LOSING WEIGHT

People who begin low-fat, vegan diets typically lose weight easily. In our research studies, the average rate is about half a kilogram (1 pound) per week. Some lose more quickly, others a bit more slowly, but half a kilogram (1 pound) a week is a good pace. If you think about what this means over a year's time, the result is impressive, particularly since you are free of the yo-yo syndrome that comes with diets based on calorie restrictions. Because this is not a short-term, starve-yourself-thin diet, it does not cause hunger, so there is no rebound bingeing. Gradual, healthy weight loss is what you can expect. Sometimes losing weight can be a bit like following the stock market. There are fluctuations up and down but the trend should be clear. If you are not losing weight, it is time to take action. Here are the steps to take.

Get back to the basics. Be sure you are following the guidelines in Chapter 4 and giving it 100 per cent. That means no animal products in your diet at all. If your diet includes fish or cheese, for example, your weight-loss efforts will be hampered.

Check for hidden oils. Packaged foods should include no more than 2 to 3 grams of fat per serving. If you frequently eat at restaurants, try to assess to what extent they are packing oils into their meals. If you are unsure, ask for foods to be steamed rather than fried or sautéed and that any sauces or dressings be served on the side. See Chapter 8.

Do a Quick Fibre Check. If you check your fibre intake (see page 107) and find that you are eating less than 40 grams of fibre per day, you'll want to bring in more beans, vegetables and fruits.

If your diet is vegan, low in fat and high in fibre, it is very hard not to lose weight. Even so, here are a few things to consider.

Don't Get Sidetracked by Rationalizations

Sometimes people who are not losing weight blame genetics, lack of exercise or something else for their problem. Genetics and exercise do play roles, of course. But if you are not losing weight, the problem is nearly always dietary.

Once, en route from Washington to London, I was busily typing away on my laptop, writing an article about diet changes for weight loss. The passenger next to me happened to see what I was typing and took an interest in the topic. He had been overweight for several years and wanted to see what I might suggest. I explained our research findings about how diet changes could cause lasting weight loss. I pointed out that the key seemed to be changing the types of foods we eat. I launched into a discussion of the benefits of vegetables, fruits, beans and whole grains and the wonderful meals they can become.

'That's interesting,' he said, 'but I think I just need to exercise more. That's my real problem. I used to exercise a lot, but lately, I've been so busy.' He brushed aside the whole topic of food.

A few minutes later, the flight attendant came by with the meal service. She served him a ham and cheese sandwich, a bag of crisps and a soft drink, which he shovelled into his mouth without a word. I suspect he did not realize that it would take a very long session at the gym to burn away those unnecessary calories. The airline also served vegetarian meals, which would have been a much better choice.

Shortly thereafter, I was talking to a patient with another doctor, Stanley Talpers, of the George Washington University School of Medicine in Washington, D.C. The patient said he hadn't been losing weight, and he figured that he just needed to walk more. Dr Talpers encouraged him to get his diet in order first because, he said, 'To lose a pound by walking, you'd have to walk to Baltimore.' It is true. Exercise is beneficial and I strongly recommend it. But a lack of exercise is not the primary reason for weight problems, and exercise can never take the place of a healthy diet.

Simplify. It pays to choose simple foods rather than processed food products. The fewer ingredients, the better – one is ideal. Beans, broccoli, carrots or brown rice, for example, do not need an ingredients list, because what you see is exactly what you get. You know that no one has added any oil or processed away any fibre.

Add more raw foods. Some people have had remarkable weight loss as a result of increasing their intake of raw foods. Chopped vegetables, salads, fresh fruit – these are all rich in fibre, with no added fat and low GIs.

BLOOD GLUCOSE NOT COMING UNDER CONTROL QUICKLY ENOUGH

The primary way of tracking your glucose control is with the HbA1c. As you know, the UK goal is to have your HbA1c under 7 per cent, but many doctors now push for even lower goals: 6.5 or 6.0 per cent. If you are not making good progress towards your goal, here are some points to consider.

Get back to the basics (again). If you are overweight, weight loss is the strongest predictor of a healthy drop in HbA1c. To jump-start weight loss, take a look at the tips above and in Chapter 6. Whether you are overweight or not, those same points are also the keys to bringing your glucose under control.

If your diet is vegan, it has no animal fat in it, of course. And if you are setting aside vegetable oils, it has very little of any kind of fat. With these healthy changes, you can just imagine those little bits of fat inside your muscle cells starting to shrivel up. As you saw in Chapter 2, these are the bits of fat that appear to be the cause of insulin resistance.

Embrace healthy carbohydrates. Many people tie one arm behind their backs by avoiding starchy foods. They imagine that beans, lentils or pasta will push their blood glucose upwards. And, of course, if you check your blood glucose after just about any meal, it will be higher than it was before. However, don't let this turn you against starchy foods and back towards fatty or high-protein foods. Here is why.

The fat in fish and chicken will tend to arrest your weight loss. It will also tend to aggravate your insulin resistance. Here is what happens in a typical case.

A man has heard that 'carbs are bad' or perhaps notices that his blood glucose has gone up briefly after a meal of rice or starchy vegetables. He decides to avoid carbohydrates and adds fish and chicken back into his diet. At first, it seems like a good change. His blood glucose does not spike strongly after meals because there is very little starch in his meals to provide glucose. 'Aha!' he says. 'I've found the diet to keep my blood sugar down!' Over the next several days, however, he notices that his fasting blood glucose values are heading in the wrong direction. They go up bit by bit, and after a week or two, the rise is significant. 'Now what?' he thinks. This is what is going on.

There are only three sources of calories: carbohydrate, fat and protein. In avoiding carbohydrate, he was left with fat – which tends to increase insulin resistance – and protein, which has problems of its own. The increased fat intake did not increase his blood glucose immediately, but fatty diets tend to increase the amount of fat inside the cells. The result is that insulin resistance gradually worsens. That means that any carbohydrate he ate later would cause a bigger blood sugar spike than it otherwise would have. As the days went by, his blood sugar gradually increased.

The answer is to avoid fatty foods and choose healthy, carbohydrate-rich foods, letting the glycaemic index help you choose the best of them (see Chapter 4). This means pulses (beans, peas and lentils), vegetables, fruits and whole grains.

Meals will always cause a temporary rise in blood glucose; what you are looking for is an overall trend downwards as your insulin sensitivity gradually improves.

See your doctor. A very common reason for rising blood glucose levels is infection. A cold, a urinary tract infection, a foot sore, an ear infection – you name it. They all tend to raise your blood glucose. Sometimes a surprisingly small cut or a cough you're hardly aware of boosts your fasting blood sugar values. As the infection heals (with medical treatment as needed), your blood glucose will recover. Your doctor may decide to adjust your diabetes medications in the interim.

Check your stress level. Stress raises blood sugar. The fight-or-flight response – the physical reaction that gets you ready to fight or run away from danger – can kick in with any sort of threat, real or imagined. A rise in blood sugar was much more useful when the threats we encountered were predators and warring tribes. That extra blood sugar fuelled the major muscle groups needed to run or fight. Today, we are more likely to be threatened by job worries, financial difficulties or relationship problems, and rising blood sugar doesn't help during those times. But stress still evokes the response and it still causes a blood sugar spike.

If stress is temporary, you will see your glucose spike resolve quickly. If stress is ongoing, get help. Meditation, yoga and other techniques can help you deal with stress. If the problem is deeper – if you are headed into depression or chronic anxiety – do not try to be a hero. See a qualified mental health professional and get started with a treatment that works for you.

Exercise. If you are sedentary, now is the time to bring physical activity into your life. Vigorous exercise helps reduce blood glucose levels. See Chapter 11.

In most cases, these steps will help bring your blood sugar down. If it remains high despite your best efforts, your doctor will want to adjust your medications.

PERSISTENT HUNGER

If you are cutting back on calories in an effort to lose weight, you may be left feeling hungry. One of the reasons I recommend a low-fat, vegan diet is that it is so substantial – it provides plenty of fibre to fill you up and has no limits on portion sizes or calories. The result is weight loss without hunger. In our research studies, we use a questionnaire to measure hunger along the way, and we consistently find that this diet leaves people feeling satisfied.

What if your meals don't quite satisfy you, though? Here are some suggestions, starting with the obvious one.

Eat more. Maybe that little bowl of oats is just not enough. When you are just getting to know new foods, it takes a little time to figure out the right serving sizes. You will soon sort this out.

Go low GI and high fibre. If you have instant oats for breakfast, you will get hungry sooner than if you have old-fashioned porridge. The difference is simply that instant oats have had their fibre sliced up. Instead of flat rolled oats, you have a box full of oat powder. That means that they cook quicker but also that they digest quicker, spike your blood sugar quicker (that is, they have a higher GI) and leave you hungry quicker. Eating foods that are in as natural a state as possible prevents that overly rapid digestion and helps keep hunger at bay.

You want foods that have both a low GI *and* high fibre content. A food that offers one doesn't necessarily have the other. For example, wholemeal bread has lots of fibre, but something about the wheat grain causes it to release its natural sugars into the bloodstream rather quickly (i.e., it has a high GI). In fact, white bread (which has had its fibre removed) has virtually the same GI as wholemeal. In contrast, rye bread digests more slowly, releasing its natural sugars into the bloodstream more gradually, which means it has a low GI. To check your fibre intake, do a Quick Fibre Check (see page 107).

Have healthy snacks. There will be many times when you will want to have a bite to eat between meals, and you should! See Chapter 5 for a discussion of the best choices.

QUIETING CRAVINGS

If you have had diabetes for any length of time, you have already been coping with the ubiquitous nature of junk food. Unhealthy snacks are everywhere. But why do they call to us as they do? Why is sugar or chocolate sometimes so attractive? Why is cheese or meat sometimes hard to resist? Where do cravings come from?

One of our research participants once asked me what was wrong with her. She had had diabetes for 12 years, and even though she knew that she should stay away from sugary foods, she craved them. Especially when she was stressed or tired, cakes, chocolate and pastries seemed to call her name. She had the cravings nearly every day. 'I think I'm just a weak-willed person,' she said. She was embarrassed about her cravings and found herself avoiding the subject when she spoke to her dietitian.

Here is the most important thing to understand about cravings: they are not caused by weak will or gluttony. Cravings are triggered by *biological properties of the foods themselves.* That is, certain foods have chemical makeups that cause us to crave them in very much the same way that drugs, alcohol and tobacco have addictive components.

Let me be clear: only certain foods lend themselves to cravings. The same foods are alluring to almost everyone.

Four types of foods trigger biochemical effects not unlike those of addictive drugs. They are not as strong or as dangerous as drugs, but the chemistry of addiction does seem to be at work with these foods. I have described these effects in detail in a book called *Breaking the Food Seduction*. Here, I will summarize the main points you need to know. The four categories of addictive food are sugar, chocolate, cheese and meat.

Sugar. Sugar is not simply sweet. In addition to its taste, it also has a mild drug-like effect. That is, it affects the brain in essentially the same way as opiate drugs – morphine and heroin, for example – albeit not as strongly. This effect helps explain why people crave sugar, especially during times of stress.

How do we know that sugar has this effect? In controlled studies, researchers use a medication called naloxone as a research tool. Naloxone is normally used in an emergency to block the effects of heroin or other opiates. If a person has overdosed on heroin, doctors inject naloxone, which blocks the heroin (and any other narcotic) from attaching to receptors in the brain. A comatose drug addict, previously on the verge of death, rapidly awakens with a dose of naloxone.

Researchers have given naloxone to volunteers and offered them various sugary foods. They then measured how much the volunteers ate and compared the results to those of the same test done without naloxone.

It turns out that naloxone causes a noticeable drop in sugar cravings. Normally, you might long for a glazed doughnut or piece of gooey cake, but with a dose of naloxone, much of the attraction is gone. The effect is particularly clear for foods that contain both sugar and fat: biscuits, cakes and ice cream.

Naloxone is given intravenously and is not a treatment for food addiction; it is a research tool. These experiments show that sugar does not simply delight the taste buds; it also stimulates the release of opiate chemicals in the brain. Just as intense exercise causes the release of endorphins – natural feel-good chemicals within the brain – sugar seems to do something very similar.

Let me be clear about this: sugar does not contain opiates. Rather, the taste of sugar on the tongue is what apparently triggers the release of opiates within the brain. In turn, these opiates trigger the release of another natural chemical, called dopamine, which is the key to the brain's pleasure centres. Drugs of abuse – heroin, cocaine, marijuana, tobacco, alcohol and all others – trigger dopamine release. Sugar appears to do the same. Evidence suggests that the effects of sugar on the brain ease pain and discomfort and give us a little boost. No wonder we turn to sugary foods, especially when we're stressed.

Sugar has the same effects on infants just a few hours old. When babies are given a heel-prick to draw a blood sample, they cry noticeably less if a bit of sugar water is dribbled into their mouth first.

Sugar cravings go beyond plain sugar itself. Some people also crave foods such as white bread or bagels, which turn to sugar rapidly and release sugar into the bloodstream. In essence, they crave high-GI foods – sugar, biscuits, crackers, white bread, potatoes or cold cereals. While we also enjoy low-GI foods, we tend not to crave them.

Chocolate. Chocolate's addictive qualities have long been recognized in psychiatric journals. In scientific studies, the most ardent chocoholics' desire falls away when they are treated with opiate-blocking drugs. These experiments show that it is not simply taste or mouthfeel that keeps us hooked. Chocolate also appears to have mild effects on our brains.

Chocolate's attraction is not due simply to its sweetness. After all, no true chocolate lover would be satisfied with sugar alone. Chocolate also contains caffeine, theobromine and phenylethylamine. These are all stimulants and they may play a role in chocolate's seduction, aside from its opiate effects.

If you are a chocolate lover, you probably already know that chocolate is sometimes more than a food: you don't just feel you *want* it, you feel you *need it*. Regrettably, chocolate carries not only a load of sugar but also a considerable load of fat.

Cheese. Yes, it may smell a bit like old socks, but cheese is one of the foods that people who are trying to improve their diets have the most trouble leaving behind. There is obviously something besides fat and cholesterol in cheese that accounts for its popularity.

That 'something' may be the dairy protein, or casein. Like all proteins, casein's molecular structure is very much like a long string of beads, with each bead being an amino acid. Normally, when proteins are digested, these amino acids come apart one by one and are absorbed into the bloodstream to be used to build body tissues and repair any damage to your body.

Casein behaves differently. As it breaks apart, it does not simply release individual amino acids. It breaks into short strings of amino acids – strings of perhaps four, five or seven 'beads'. They are not just the amino acid building blocks for protein; they are also biologically active compounds with a mild narcotic action. Scientists call them casomorphins – casein-derived morphine-like compounds. If scientists were to feed you cheese and then take a sample of your digestive tract contents, they would find an array of casomorphins with mild narcotic actions. Some have speculated that the narcotic effects of casomorphins are responsible for cheese's attraction. These effects may also explain why cheese can be constipating, since narcotic compounds often slow digestion.

Scientists are still trying to understand casomorphins. We know that they form in the digestive tract as casein breaks apart and that they can pass into the bloodstream of nursing infants. They seem to act as mild sedatives for babies. We also know that casein is present in milk and ice cream and is especially concentrated in cheese. What we do not yet know is how extensively the casomorphins are absorbed into the bloodstream of adults.

By now you know if cheese is your thing. If so, its fat and cholesterol contents are conspiring against you. Shortly, we will look at how to kick this and other food addictions.

Meat. Men, in particular, often describe meat as the very last food they would ever want to give up. No matter how often they are reminded of what it is doing to their waistline or cholesterol test results, many have trouble breaking their emotional attachment to roast beef, steak or chicken wings.

Once again, experiments with opiate-blocking drugs suggest that part of the desire for meat may have its basis in opiate effects within the brain. Researchers in England gave opiate-blocking drugs to volunteers and tested their desire for ham, salami and tuna. The results showed that when the opiate effects were blocked, volunteers lost much of their interest in meat.[1]

Resetting Your Priorities

If cravings are sabotaging your new food programme, take heart. You are not a glutton or the victim of a bad upbringing. The fact is, you are not attracted to just any food, or even to most foods. You may like apples, oranges, bananas or asparagus, but you have never once turned to them for solace during moments of stress. You have never raced off to the supermarket because you just *had* to have cauliflower. You have turned to sugar, chocolate, cheese or meat because these are more than mere foods. They have chemical effects on the brain. Some beverages, such as wine or coffee, also have drug-like effects and can be addictive. But as far as foods go, those four comprise the whole list. These foods work their unfortunate magic on just about everyone.

Before we see what you might eat instead of that sugary doughnut, chocolate bar or cheeseburger, let's look again at what happens inside your brain when you eat these foods.

A network of cells deep inside the brain makes up what is sometimes called your pleasure centre. Indeed, it is responsible for feelings of pleasure. Without it, life would be one big grey day.

The pleasure centre is not there just for fun, however. It is there to keep you alive and to maintain the species. Here is why: if you got absolutely no pleasure from eating, you would have no motivation to eat. You might forget about foods entirely! Likewise, if sex were a total bore, the species would soon die out. Thus, when you eat or have sex, your pleasure centre gives you a little bit of dopamine as a kind of reward.

In the process, that dopamine release causes slight neurological changes, changes that put high-priority status on repeating whatever you have just done. 'That was fun,' your pleasure centre seems to say. 'Let's make sure we do that again.'

In nature, this would mean getting a reward for finding a new food source or a receptive mate, with the result that you would take advantage of your find again and again. The problem is that this system is easily hijacked. Alcohol, recreational drugs, tobacco – and yes, unhealthy foods – cause significant dopamine release, so not only do you like them, you also want to have them again and again. Your pleasure centre rearranges your priorities to favour whatever stimulated it most recently. You find yourself planning your day around sugar or chocolate, just as an alcoholic might regularly think about where the next drink is coming from. If you have ever wondered why these otherwise banal foods have such sway, it is because they hijack your brain's pleasure circuitry and your internal priority-setting system.

Breaking Free

If the occasional taste of sugar or chocolate is really not a big part of your life, there is no need to worry about it. But if your waistline is expanding before your very eyes, or your health is suffering from your food habits, it is time to wake up and smell the addiction. What do you do if you're hooked?

The best way to deal with unhealthy foods is to avoid teasing yourself. Set them aside completely, at least for now. Do not keep them in the house and do not buy them. There is no need to worry about whether you will return to them in the future. For now, just leave them alone.

In the process, your brain's priorities can return to what really is good for you. You are likely to find that your desire for unhealthy foods fades the longer you are away from them. The following steps will also help.

- Eat a healthy breakfast and don't skip meals. Cravings kick in when you are hungry.

- Get regular exercise so you're tired enough to sleep soundly and be sure to get plenty of rest. Cravings are stronger when you are not sleeping well.

- Avoid situations that trigger cravings. Some people find that their cravings are triggered by being alone, by television cooking shows, by concession stands at film theatres, or by certain friends who are preoccupied with food problems of their own. Try to identify your triggers and eliminate them as much as possible.

Getting the Taste without the Regrets

Sometimes a simple substitution can help you steer away from an unhealthy food. Here are a few.

If you crave sugar: In recipes, maple syrup, molasses and granulated sugarcane juice (Sucanat) can sometimes substitute for table sugar. These are hardly health foods! The idea is to replace refined white sugar with a smaller amount of syrup or juice. They're so flavourful you won't notice you're using less.

Sucralose (Splenda) is a calorie-free sweetener made from cane sugar to which chlorine has been chemically added, greatly increasing the sweetness of the final product. Sugar alcohols, such as mannitol, sorbitol and xylitol, are low-calorie sweeteners sometimes used in sweets, chewing gum and desserts. They have about half the calories of table sugar. There are, of course, other artificial sweeteners. The disadvantage of the lot of them is that they do not help you break your love affair with sweets, so when artificial sweeteners are not available, you will find yourself returning to sugar.

My friend and colleague Dr Hans Diehl, head of the pioneering Coronary Health Improvement Project in the US, says the best thing to do for a sweet tooth is to 'have it pulled!' The idea is that if you set sweets aside, you will eventually just forget about them.

Of course, the best choices are fresh fruits – nature's own sweet foods. It also helps to make sure your diet contains an adequate amount of complex carbohydrate – grains, sweet potatoes and beans, for example. These foods provide the energy you need in a form that is much more healthy than sugar.

If you crave chocolate: Cocoa powder is essentially defatted chocolate. It can be used in beverages and baking or turned into a dip for strawberries or other fresh fruit. You can also find low-fat frozen ice cream substitutes made from soya, as well as sorbets.

If you crave cheese: Get to know nutritional yeast. Sold in the supplement aisle of health food stores, nutritional yeast flakes (not brewer's or baker's yeast) add a cheese-like flavour to sauces and casseroles.

In recipes, you can replace ricotta or cottage cheese with mashed, water-packed tofu mixed with a little lemon juice. If you're choosing soya cheeses, read the label to check the fat content and to see whether they're made with added casein, the dairy protein.

If you crave meat: Good substitutes for burgers and cold meats are now widely available. Tofu, tempeh and textured vegetable protein are versatile products that substitute well for meat in recipes. See the Menus and Recipes section of this book for many ideas. Surprisingly enough, the desire for meat fades very rapidly once it is removed from the diet. People who thought they could not live without steak or a salmon fillet soon find they have absolutely no desire for it.

Genetic Influences on Cravings

Although cravings can affect anyone, some people may be especially vulnerable. Researchers have found that some people are born with fewer receptors for dopamine, the brain chemical responsible for pleasurable feelings. Apparently, this lack means that they get less dopamine stimulation and less of the feel-good sensation that dopamine provides. This leaves them feeling a bit out of sorts compared to other people. As a result, they are drawn to tobacco, alcohol or drugs; presumably, they are seeking the stimulation that nature has not given them. They may even fall prey to compulsive gambling or compulsive eating.

It all starts with a gene. The receptors for dopamine are built according to the specifications on your chromosomes – the long spiral staircase–shaped strings of genes in each of your cells that determine who you are. Your mother and father passed along their genes to you, and the makeup of your body reflects the combination of the two. If either parent passed along a gene for having too few dopamine receptors, you would have roughly one-third fewer receptors than other people.

If you were able to sample individuals in smoking cessation programmes or drug treatment clinics, you would find that as many as 40 per cent have a gene that causes them to have too few receptors called dopamine receptor D2, or DRD2 for short.

Several years ago, I found myself wondering if people who have trouble following a healthy diet may have this genetic variation. Dr Ernest Noble, of the University of California, Los Angeles, conducted genetic analyses on our patients. To our surprise, he found that nearly half of our research participants with type 2 diabetes had the gene that was associated with fewer than normal dopamine receptors. That is far higher than the roughly one-in-five prevalence in the general population.

This raised a disturbing question: did the lack of dopamine receptors lead them to overeat? Did overeating then lead to weight gain, which in turn triggered diabetes? We have not yet sorted all this out, but we did find that while people with this gene improved a great deal on our diet, they got somewhat less benefit compared to those with the normal number of dopamine receptors. Their HbA1c values dropped by about 0.9 percentage point on average, compared to a drop of 1.6 points for those without the gene. Could this gene mean some people are born with less resistance to the temptations of unhealthy foods? Or is there perhaps some direct biochemical effect of a lack of dopamine? Does less dopamine equal greater insulin resistance? We do not yet know.

At present, this type of genetic testing is done only in research studies. Your doctor cannot determine whether you are genetically endowed with fewer dopamine receptors. In fact, as far as your food

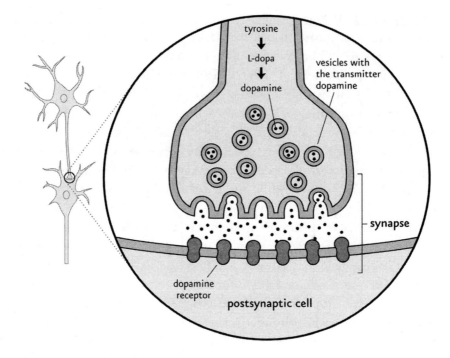

tyrosine

L-dopa

dopamine

vesicles with
the transmitter
dopamine

synapse

dopamine
receptor

postsynaptic cell

The brain cell at the top contains small packets (vesicles) of dopamine. When you experience a pleasurable sensation, these vesicles release their dopamine into the space (synapse) that lies between that cell and the next one. As the dopamine molecules reach the next cell, they attach to its dopamine receptors, and their effect depends on how many dopamine receptors you have. Some people have approximately one-third fewer receptors than other people.

plan is concerned, it does not matter. Regardless of your genetic makeup, the diet described in this book is very likely to help you. I raise the issue of genetics simply to underscore the point that cravings and food addictions are *physical*, not moral issues. They are due to the properties of foods themselves that interact with our natural biochemistry.

One final point: if certain foods act like drugs, it pays to treat them like drugs. In other words, avoid them. Just as it is harder for a smoker to cut down than to quit and harder for an alcoholic to drink wine moderately than to quit drinking altogether, it is very tough to tease yourself with foods that have you in their clutches. It is actually easier to leave them alone completely and do your best to forget about them. If you have not had one of these biochemically active foods in a few weeks, you crave it much less than you would if you had it yesterday.

DIGESTIVE PROBLEMS

A plant-based diet is great for people who have been bothered by constipation. Its natural fibre is what your digestive tract needs. Some foods can cause a bit of wind, however. If you experience this, here is what to do about it.

First, only certain foods cause wind. Grains, fruits and most vegetables get a not-guilty verdict. Beans and undercooked cruciferous vegetables (broccoli, cabbage, cauliflower and brussels sprouts, for example) are the main culprits. Chances are, all you need to do is have smaller servings. If you have been replacing a huge steak with a huge plate of beans, remember that a small amount of beans goes a long way. Try downsizing your portions.

Over time, you will find that your body adjusts, so you can have larger portions with less wind. If you cook beans from scratch, be sure to discard the water used to soak them and then cook them in fresh water. Cook them well (there are no *al dente* beans)! The same goes for cruciferous vegetables. Yes, we all love a stalk of fresh broccoli from the crudités tray, but if that gives you digestive trouble, cook vegetables until you can easily pierce them with a fork.

It goes without saying that you want to avoid dairy products and sugar. Dairy products, of course, are already off the list, but digestive problems are yet another reason to steer clear of them, as you saw in Chapter 4. The lactose (milk sugar) that makes up a large percentage of the calories in skimmed milk causes many people to have wind, cramps and diarrhoea. Here is why.

During infancy, the lactase enzyme is produced within the body and breaks lactose apart in the baby's intestinal tract so it can be absorbed and used for energy. As children leave infancy behind, however, most lose this enzyme. The result, lactose intolerance, was once thought to be abnormal, but it is now known to be the biological norm, not only for humans but for all mammals. Because the body's lactase production tails off gradually, many people do not make the connection between their digestive symptoms and milk products.

In about 85 per cent of Caucasians, a genetic mutation causes the lactase enzyme to persist well into adulthood. Even so, lactose intolerance will eventually affect many of them, too. Cutting out dairy products for a few days will show you whether you are among them.

Some adults have trouble digesting table sugar (sucrose). Once again, it is easy to check. Simply set it aside for a few days and see if your symptoms improve.

HIGH TRIGLYCERIDES

When your doctor checks your cholesterol, triglycerides will also be listed on the laboratory report. Triglycerides are molecules of fat that are transported in the blood for various purposes. As with cholesterol, having a certain amount of triglycerides in the blood is a normal part of human biochemistry. However, when triglycerides are high, they increase the risk of heart problems, diseases of the pancreas and other problems. As you saw in Chapter 7, a normal triglyceride concentration is less than 1.7 mmol/l. Values between 1.7 and 2.2 mmol/l are considered borderline, and values of 2.2 to 5.5 mmol/l are high. Concentrations of above 5.5 mmol/l are considered very high.

Some studies have suggested that diets high in refined carbohydrates may cause a temporary rise in triglycerides. High-fibre and low-GI foods appear to have the opposite effect.[2] You will want to make a special point of favouring these foods. In addition, a low-fat, vegan diet helps you lose weight, which in turn reduces triglycerides.

Regular exercise helps, too. Moderate physical activity, such as walking, lowers triglyceride concentrations by an average of 0.1 mmol/l, and more strenuous activity can have greater effects.[3] You will also benefit by avoiding alcohol. Alcohol appears to raise triglycerides slightly, so when you avoid it, triglycerides slide back down.[4,5]

INTERACTION BETWEEN VEGETABLES AND PRESCRIPTION BLOOD THINNERS

Warfarin (Coumadin) is a blood thinner prescribed to prevent heart attacks, strokes, blood clots in the legs and other problems. It acts by antagonizing the effects of vitamin K, which is involved in building the proteins your body uses in the clotting process.

Many people taking warfarin believe they have to avoid vegetables, especially green leafy vegetables, that are rich in vitamin K because the vitamin will affect the formation of clots. But avoiding these healthy foods would leave them very low in important vitamins and minerals.

I encourage you to discuss this issue with your doctor and your dietitian, but the answer is not to avoid vegetables. What matters is maintaining a fairly steady amount of them in your diet so your warfarin dosage does not need to be continually adjusted. If you eat lots of healthy vegetables and then suddenly stop, warfarin's actions become stronger, increasing the risk of bleeding. On the other hand, if you were to generally avoid vegetables and one day suddenly increase your intake, the vitamin K in these foods would have the opposite effect, making it easier for your body to form clots. Bottom line: enjoy vegetables and keep the amount fairly constant from day to day.

By the way, alcohol increases warfarin's effects, which is why doctors encourage people taking it to avoid alcohol. Many medications (e.g., aspirin, paracetamol and many others) can also accentuate warfarin's action.

If you have hit any bumps in the road, I hope you have found these suggestions helpful and that you are now back on track with a healthy diet.

CHAPTER 10

Which Supplements Should You Take?

News stories and advertisements trumpet the benefits of various nutritional supplements. Chemists and health food shops are stocked with shelf after shelf of them. Which ones help and which ones are unnecessary?

Here is some basic information that will help you decide. You should, however, talk to your doctor, pharmacist or dietitian about which products you may take. You may have a particular need for one or another supplement depending on your health. Or you may need to avoid certain products because they interfere with medications you are taking.

If you are adding supplements that might affect your blood sugar, be sure to check your blood glucose regularly. Refer to Chapter 7 for how to recognize and treat low blood sugar.

Let's look at specific vitamins and other nutritional compounds, starting with the basics.

Multivitamin. Taking a multivitamin is a good idea for a few reasons.

First, it provides vitamin B_{12}, which you need for healthy blood and nerves. Yes, you can find vitamin B_{12} in some fortified products, such as breakfast cereals and soya milk, but most sources are animal derived and supply unwanted cholesterol and fat. Many people, particularly older people, tend to run low on vitamin B_{12} regardless of their diets, perhaps because their bodies become less efficient at absorbing it. A daily multivitamin keeps you covered in a healthy way.

Second, a multivitamin provides vitamin D. Your body normally produces this vitamin when sunlight hits your skin. But if you are indoors most of the day, you may be missing the natural source, and a multivitamin can make up for that. Vitamin D helps your body absorb calcium and has important anticancer properties.

Third, multivitamins contain folic acid. While this B vitamin is known for helping prevent birth defects, it also appears to have an anti-cancer effect.

In June 2002, a report in the *Journal of the American Medical Association* recommended taking a multivitamin not just once a day but twice, to ensure adequate amounts of vitamins B_{12} and D.[1] For women attempting to conceive, a multivitamin plus a 400-microgram folic acid supplement is recommended.

For adults, it is a good idea to choose a multivitamin without iron because most people already have plenty of stored iron and do not need more (if you have a history of anaemia, your doctor should advise you about whether you need iron supplements). Also, choose a vegetarian formula (all health food stores carry them). It will supply vitamin A as beta-carotene rather than as preformed vitamin A, which can be toxic if you overdo it.

Sometimes meat eaters imagine that they are getting complete nutrition without a multivitamin. The fact is, they often run low on vitamin C, folic acid, beta-carotene and other nutrients. They also generally run low on fibre, but multivitamins cannot make up for a fibre deficit, nor can they counter the effects of the cholesterol, fat or other undesirables found in the animal products they are eating.

Vitamin B_{12}. This vitamin is essential for healthy blood cells and nerve function. If you do not take a daily multivitamin, you should take a vitamin B_{12} supplement that provides at least 5 micrograms. Nearly all brands contain more than this, but higher doses are not toxic.

Vitamin D. As noted above, vitamin D is produced as a result of your skin being exposed to sunlight. It helps you absorb calcium, among other functions. It is a good idea to spend 15 to 20 minutes daily outdoors. If you get this sun exposure, there is no need for dietary supplementation. If you do not and also do not take a regular multivitamin, a 400-IU vitamin D supplement is a good idea.

Aside from the basic vitamins, some other supplements have shown promise for people with diabetes.

Cinnamon. Cinnamon has been shown to cut fasting glucose levels by 18 to 29 per cent. As little as ½ teaspoon of ordinary cinnamon added to your morning oats or other foods not only seems to reduce blood sugar, but also appears to reduce blood cholesterol levels.[2] Some of cinnamon's helpful effects may be explained by compounds called polyphenol polymers, which are found in the spice and have an insulin-like action.[3]

Magnesium. In Harvard's Nurses' Health Study, women who had more magnesium in their diets had a significantly lower likelihood of developing diabetes.[4] Apparently, magnesium increases insulin sensitivity and may increase the secretion of insulin from the pancreas, which suggests that it may also be helpful after diabetes has been diagnosed.

This does not mean, however, that you need a magnesium supplement. Foods rich in magnesium include whole grains (grains with their natural fibre intact) such as brown rice, barley and oats, as well as green vegetables such as spinach and Swiss chard. Many bean varieties are also rich in magnesium. In the Harvard study, a 'high' intake was about 400 milligrams per day. The chart on the opposite page shows the magnesium content of many common foods.

Chromium. Chromium is an element that helps insulin work better, meaning that it helps the hormone escort glucose from your bloodstream into your cells. It is naturally present in many foods, such as broccoli, green beans, whole grains, nuts and even coffee. Some experts recommend taking supplements as well. Whether that is a good idea for you depends on how much of these chromium-rich foods you eat regularly.

Technically speaking, chromium is what is called an insulin cofactor – an insulin helper, if you will. In the same way that you cannot use a jack to lift your car if its handle is missing, insulin has trouble bringing glucose into cells without chromium to help it work properly.

Chromium's essential role was discovered only relatively recently. In the late 1960s, researchers found that chromium deficiency could lead to high blood sugar levels.[5] In 1977, Canadian researchers described the case of a woman in her mid-thirties who was receiving all her nutrition intravenously following intestinal surgery. As time went by, she began to lose weight. Her blood sugar started to rise inexplicably, and eventually, she developed nerve symptoms in her legs that appeared to be diabetic neuropathy. Her doctors had to administer large insulin doses

Magnesium Content of Common Foods		
FOOD	PORTION	MAGNESIUM (MG)
Broccoli	1 cup (90 g), boiled	38
Brown rice	1 cup (200 g), boiled	86
Brussels sprouts	8	32
Chickpeas, canned	1 cup (240 g)	78
Dates, dried	10 medium	29
Figs, dried	10 medium	111
Green beans	1 cup (125 g), boiled	32
Kale	1 cup (125 g), boiled	24
Lentils	1 cup (200 g), boiled	71
Butter beans	1 cup (180 g), boiled	82
Haricot beans	1 cup (180 g), boiled	107
Oats, instant	2 packets, cooked	70
Peas	1 cup (160 g), boiled	62
Raisins	⅔ cup (100 g)	35
Soyabeans	1 cup (180 g), boiled	148
Spinach	1 cup (180 g), boiled	158
Sweet potato	1 cup (320 g), boiled	32
Tofu	½ cup (125 g)	118
White beans	1 cup (180 g), boiled	113

ADAPTED FROM: Jean A.T. Pennington and Judith S. Douglass. *Bowes and Church's Food Values of Portions Commonly Used.* 18th edition. Lippincott Williams and Wilkins, 2005.

to bring her blood sugar under control. Eventually, they gave her chromium, which had been absent from her feeding formula. In just a few weeks, her blood glucose fell to the point where she no longer required insulin and her nerve symptoms disappeared.[6]

Although correcting chromium deficiencies is essential for blood glucose control, it is not yet clear whether adding extra chromium helps, or if it is safe to do so. Studies in which researchers gave chromium to people with type 1, type 2 or gestational diabetes have yielded mixed results. The problem may be that some studies were small and used rather small chromium doses, but some studies using higher doses (up to 1,000 micrograms) in individuals with type 2 diabetes have shown no benefit.[7] As a result, most diabetes authorities do not recommend chromium supplements.[8,9]

International standards suggest that the safe and adequate daily intakes of chromium for adults aged 19 to 50 are 35 micrograms for men and 25 micrograms for women. For people over 50, the amounts are 30 micrograms for men and 20 micrograms for women. Here is the amount of chromium found in some common foods.

Chromium Content of Common Foods		
FOOD	**PORTION**	**CHROMIUM (MCG)**
Broccoli	½ cup (45 g), cooked	11
Grape juice	1 cup (240 ml)	8
English muffin, wholemeal	1	4
Potatoes, mashed	1 cup (210 g), cooked	3
Garlic, dried	1 teaspoon	3
Basil, dried	1 tablespoon	2
Orange juice	1 cup (240 ml)	2
Wholemeal bread	2 slices	2
Red wine	5 fl oz (150 ml)	1–13
Apple, with skin	1 medium	1
Banana	1 medium	1
Green beans	½ cup (60 g), cooked	1

ADAPTED FROM: National Institutes of Health, http://ods.od.nih.gov/factsheets/Chromium_pf.asp#h2, accessed December 16, 2005.

While you are making sure to include chromium-rich foods in your menu, it may also help to steer clear of sugar and refined grain products such as white flour. These foods are not only low in chromium, they also increase chromium loss from the body. Loss of the mineral is also increased by the stresses of infection, strenuous exercise and pregnancy.

If you are going to supplement, you should be aware that chromium is included in most common multivitamins, usually in amounts ranging from 100 to 200 micrograms, so additional supplementation may not be necessary.

The safety of high chromium doses has not been as extensively studied as that of other minerals. Studies using chromium for diabetes treatment often exceed the amounts recommended by the US government, using doses of up to 1,000 micrograms per day. Individuals with impaired liver or kidney function may be at risk for adverse effects and should probably stay well below this level. The long-term benefits and risks of chromium supplementation are not known.

Most typical multivitamins easily provide you with adequate chromium. If you choose to take higher amounts, it is a good idea to check with your doctor first.

Alpha-lipoic acid. Alpha-lipoic acid, sometimes called thioctic acid, is naturally produced in the human body. It plays important roles in the mitochondria, the microscopic 'burners' that provide energy in the cells. It works as a cofactor for several enzymes related to energy metabolism.

Supplemental alpha-lipoic acid is used not to counteract deficiencies but to act essentially like a drug. In high doses, it acts as an antioxidant. In people with type 2 diabetes, it appears to increase insulin sensitivity and reduce symptoms of nerve damage.[10,11]

In many studies of alpha-lipoic acid, researchers used intravenous infusions rather than oral doses. So far, it appears to be safe, but it is not yet clear whether it will yield clinically important effects over the long run and if so, what doses are safe and effective for long-term use.

CHAPTER 11

Exercise for the
Rest of Us

Yes, exercise is good for you. Physical activity reduces your blood sugar and is good for your heart. It improves the quality of your sleep and your overall energy level. When you get into an exercise groove, you really feel great.

For many of us, however, exercise conjures up images of 'no pain, no gain' workouts and unrewarding drudgery. Many people have trouble getting into an exercise routine; it just does not seem to work for them. For every person I hear say something like this:

> I feel so good when I exercise. I have more energy, my blood sugar comes way down and I just feel great. I can't imagine a day without it.

. . . there's another who feels more like this:

> I really just can't get into exercise. I know I'd do better if I did, but every time I join a gym or resolve to start exercising, it just doesn't last.

If you are carrying around a lot of extra weight, exercise can be difficult. Perhaps you are limited by joint pain or heart problems. Maybe your good intentions just seem to vanish when the time comes to lace up your trainers. In this chapter, we will tackle the various aspects of exercise – its benefits, its limitations and the difficulties in getting started – and see how to make it work for you.

One note of reassurance: if you cannot exercise because of a physical limitation, you can still lose weight, cut your blood sugar and live a healthy life. In fact, most of the benefits of the diet changes you have read about came *without* exercise. That is because in our diet studies, we usually ask our volunteers *not* to alter their exercise patterns, so we can isolate the effects of a diet change for research purposes. Exercise certainly adds to the health benefits that a good diet brings, but if it is simply not in the picture, you can still do well.

WHAT YOU ARE WORKING FOR

Different kinds of exercise provide very different benefits.

Aerobic exercise is any sort of rhythmic, continuous activity you perform for a sustained period – usually at least 10 minutes. Brisk walking, running, playing tennis, dancing or skating can all be aerobic. This type of exercise reduces your blood sugar and triglycerides, and if you keep it up, you will live longer.

Resistance exercise is weight lifting and other exercises in which the emphasis is on muscular effort: press-ups and deep knee bends, for example. It builds your muscle mass or at least preserves the muscle you have. It also improves insulin sensitivity.

Flexibility exercises (stretching) are intended to maintain the range of motion of your joints. They can also relieve stress.

Below, I will give you guidelines for how much and how often you should exercise.

A diet–exercise combination can help prevent diabetes from ever developing. A groundbreaking study called the Diabetes Prevention Programme followed 3,234 people whose blood sugar levels were creeping upwards but were not yet high enough to warrant a diagnosis of diabetes. With a combination of diet and exercise, the participants were able to cut the risk of developing the disease by 58 per cent. The exercise regime totalled 150 minutes per week – a half hour five times a week.[1]

There is a very big caveat with all of this, though: exercise can boost the effects of a healthy diet, but it cannot make up for a poor one. In fact, of the two components – diet and exercise – the diet portion is much more important for weight loss and ultimately for preventing or controlling diabetes.

A careful review of published research showed that people who simply began exercise programmes did not lose much more weight than people who remained sedentary.[2] Some studies are more optimistic, suggesting that an exercise programme may boost the weight-loss effect of a diet change by about 20 per cent.[3] But it is clear that for weight control, exercise cannot take the place of diet changes.

This does not mean that exercise is of no help at all. It is definitely helpful. For instance, once a person has diabetes, exercise helps reduce HbA1c. In a review of several studies testing the effect of exercise, the average HbA1c in volunteers who began exercise programmes fell to 7.7 per cent, which is better than the 8.3 per cent found in those who did not exercise.[4] Once again, however, that result pales in comparison to the benefits of a diet change. To prevent diabetes or bring it under control, it is best to use both diet *and* exercise.

One part of your body that benefits tremendously from exercise is your heart. A recent study tracked physical activity levels in adults with type 2 diabetes over a period of 19 years and looked specifically at the risk of dying of heart disease. It turned out that those who were moderately physically active were about 40 per cent less likely to succumb to heart disease than were sedentary people. Their routines included at least 4 hours per week of moderate exercise such as walking, cycling or light gardening.[5] Active people also cut their risk of stroke.[6]

There are three other exercise benefits worth noting. First, exercise and eating are mutually exclusive activities, unlike eating and watching television. It is easy to wolf down extra calories while watching your favourite crime drama or a movie, but it is a real challenge while you are playing tennis. Exercise is calorie-free fun.

Second, exercise helps you sleep. If you have given your muscles a good workout, they *demand* sleep. You will sleep much more soundly than if you had spent the entire day behind your desk, watching television or reading. And when you are well rested, it is easier to stay focused on a healthy diet and say no to unhealthy foods.

Third, exercise makes you feel better. It lifts your spirits and is a natural antidepressant.

TYPE I AND TYPE II MUSCLE CELLS

Why do some people love exercise and others loathe it? Surprisingly enough, part of the reason is genetic. If you could look inside your muscles and compare them with those of other people, you would discover a sobering fact: some people were born to exercise. That is to say, their muscles naturally contain many type I cells (the name has nothing to do with type 1 diabetes; it is just a coincidence). These muscle cells have a particularly strong blood supply made possible by a rich network of capillaries that bring in oxygen and reduce fatigue. They also have an extra supply of an enzyme called lipoprotein lipase, which breaks fats apart to be used as fuel. The result is extra energy for a long run. When you see people running down the road looking invigorated rather than haggard, or when someone waxes poetic about the joys of the runner's high, do not envy their resolve. Odds are, they were born with muscles that are just loaded with type I cells.

Other people's muscles contain mostly type II cells, which are fine for short bursts of exercise but have less endurance for the long haul.

Now, having said that, it is important to realize that muscles can change, at least to a degree. If you gradually but steadily increase the intensity of your workouts (within the limits of safety), the blood supply to type II cells increases. Eventually, they become almost as vigorous as type I cells.

I raise this biological distinction to make an important point: exercise aptitude – or lack of it – is not a question of character; it is biology at work. If you have been beating yourself up for your lack of athletic prowess, it is time for a reprieve.

MAKING IT WORK FOR YOU

There are two keys to making exercise work.

First, it is essential to keep it fun. For most of us, that means it should be a social event. It is more fun to go walking with someone else than by yourself. If you plan to exercise at a gym, you are much more likely to keep it up if you sign up for a class – aerobics, yoga or whatever – than if you go it alone. You are also much more likely to actually get to your class if someone is going with you.

You might make an occasion of it and plan an especially healthy meal afterwards. If you are going dancing or playing tennis, the word *exercise* may not even enter your mind. Your activity is too enjoyable to call it that. Keep it fun because otherwise, you will not do it twice, much less three times a week. And for most people, fun means friends. You need other people with you to make it work.

Second, it is important to exercise regularly rather than intermittently. To paraphrase Newton's first law of motion, 'an object at rest tends to stay at rest, and an object in motion tends to stay in motion'. If the object at rest is you – that is, if you are firmly planted on the couch – you will tend to stay at rest. If, on the other hand, you and a friend go for a walk every other day after dinner, you will stay on track.

There is another reason for keeping exercise regular: the effect of any single exercise session is small. If you belong to a gym, you can see this for yourself. Just jump on the nearest treadmill and run flat out for a mile. Then, as you catch your breath, push the little button that lets you see how many calories you have burned. Surprised? That's right, you have expended only about 100 calories. That's less than half the calories in an order of McDonald's french fries or a bottle of cola. A single exercise session every now and then will not help you any more than occasionally eating a healthy meal. To be really effective, healthy habits have to be part of your routine.

Also, for better or worse, exercise effects do not last very long. If you are laid up with an injury, for example, you will find your blood sugar or weight gradually returning to its pre-exercise level. People who get into a habit of going for a brisk walk or bicycle ride every day or two sustain their benefits.

Bottom line: to make exercise work, keep it fun and keep it regular.

SEE YOUR DOCTOR FIRST

Before you embark on a new exercise programme, be sure to get your doctor's okay. Is your heart up to it? Are your joints ready? How vulnerable are you to hypo- or hyperglycaemia? Do you have any special eye or foot problems that could be aggravated by exercise? Your doctor should address all of these questions.

Beware of jumping into vigorous exercise too quickly. If it has been months (or years) since you tried exercising regularly, start slowly. It takes time for your body to reap the rewards of your new, improved diet. A heart patient, for example, who begins a vegetarian diet, stops smoking and starts really taking care of himself will probably feel better very soon. His chest pain may melt away within a few weeks and he will be eager to jump into a vigorous exercise programme. The fact is, though, that he still has the artery blockages he has been accumulating for years. Yes, the damage can be reversed, but it takes time and he should not push himself past the limits set by his doctor.

If you have type 1 diabetes, you may find that your blood sugar drops precipitously during and after exercise. This can also happen to people with type 2 diabetes who use insulin or drugs that cause insulin secretion (e.g., gliclazide, glipizide, glimepiride, nateglinide or repaglinide). It is important to be alert to the possibility of a major blood sugar drop and to adjust your eating schedule, medication use and exercise accordingly.

Occasionally, the opposite can occur: you may find that your blood sugar is temporarily higher after exercise than it was before.

A research team based in Florida tracked blood glucose in children with type 1 diabetes as they walked on a treadmill in four 15-minute bouts, with 5-minute rest periods in between. Their average blood glucose was 8.8 mmol/l when they started, but it had fallen to 6.2 mmol/l afterwards. At least one-quarter of the children became hypoglycaemic during or right after the exercise. They were also more likely to be hypoglycaemic during the following night.[7]

Exercise can reduce your blood sugar and quickly. Of course, if you eat too much in an effort to prevent hypoglycaemia, your blood sugar can go too high.

For these reasons, it is important to speak with your doctor about your medication, diet and exercise programme to make sure you are ready for exercise, then make whatever adjustments are needed for safety.

GETTING STARTED

Okay. Your doctor has given you the green light, you have rustled up some friends and you are ready to begin.

If you were imagining that I would push you into hours of jogging and weight lifting and harangue you with exhortations about 'no pain, no gain' – well, push those thoughts aside. The goal is to enjoy exercise – so much so that it becomes part of your life.

For aerobic exercise, I suggest starting with a half-hour brisk walk 5 days a week, assuming that you have no health-related exercise restrictions. If you prefer, you can exercise three times per week, either taking brisk 1-hour walks or doing more vigorous half-hour workouts. You can also break up those 30-minute walks into 10- or 15-minute mini-workouts if you like. Do not allow yourself more than 2 sedentary days in a row. The benefits of walking are not as great as those of a more vigorous exercise programme, but it is a good place to start.

The important thing is to find a time that works for you. A friend tells me that if she does not get her exercise in before lunchtime, it is just not going to happen – too many unexpected demands crop up each day to count on free time in the afternoon or evening.

It is a good idea to put exercise on your schedule, as if it were an appointment with yourself, and to include someone else in your plans.

A pedometer will help you keep track of your progress. In our research studies, we use an Omron pedometer to track the total number of steps participants take each day as well as the number of 'aerobic steps' (steps taken as part of a continuous walk of at least 10 minutes). The participants can also programme in their stride length to track mileage and even estimate their calorie burn. Take note of how many (or how few!) steps you take in a normal day, then gradually increase them. For reference, 10,000 steps or more is a vigorous day for a healthy person, but you may not have the strength or stamina to do that many. Do not push beyond your doctor's recommended limits.

A podiatrist or nurse specializing in diabetes will help you take care of your feet. This is important since exercise can sometimes cause foot injuries or aggravate an existing injury. It is surprising how often people are unaware of gradually worsening foot sores.

Your doctor will help you gauge your improvement and can advise you about increasing your exercise intensity. As your endurance improves, you will find that your energy just keeps increasing, and your weight and blood sugar stay under better control.

What's Your Pleasure?

Taking a regular walk is a great way to start exercising because it's so easy to fit into your schedule. When you are ready to add other activities, think about which ones you might enjoy.

- Aerobics classes can be fun, social and sometimes intense.
- Dancing is wonderful exercise, with better music than most aerobics classes.
- Tennis, either singles or doubles, can be a great workout.
- Many health clubs organize squash or tennis lessons.
- Golf can be great exercise if you walk the course.
- Local running clubs often organize training groups for people working towards 5-K, 10-K and half- and full-marathon races.
- Libraries are a source of exercise videos and DVDs.

For resistance and flexibility exercises, I suggest that you work with a personal trainer, both for safety reasons and to individualize your programme using the right equipment. Professional athletes are not the only ones with access to professional fitness expertise; you can have it, too. A personal trainer can help you plan a full programme, not only for aerobics but also for strength training and flexibility.

Most health clubs have trainers on the staff and may even offer a free session as an incentive to join. Why not take advantage of it? If you do not plan on joining a gym, just make an appointment for a single exercise counselling session so you can get a programme that is right for you. Then schedule a follow-up.

For people with type 2 diabetes who have no health-related exercise restrictions, it is advisable to do resistance exercise that includes all major muscle groups three times a week. The workout should include three sets of 8 to 10 repetitions at a weight that cannot be lifted more than 8 to 10 times.[8]

No Blame, No Shame

With exercise, just as with diet, most people are not yet where they would like to be. Most of us do not have heart rate monitors, the latest running shoes or shorts with a pocket designed to hold an iPod.

When the subject of exercise comes up in conversation, we may be at a bit of a loss if we are not part of the gym culture. Guilt and blame come into the picture when we are sedentary, just as they do when we are not eating well. Sometimes family members try to scold us into exercising, and sometimes doctors try the same approach. But all their moralizing is nothing compared to the guilt-laden punishment we heap on ourselves, as if not exercising were a tremendous moral failing.

If that is where you are, let me encourage you to set guilt and blame aside. Just let it all go. Tell your guilt-inducing friends that up until now, you have been illustrating Newton's first law of motion. Now, however, you are about to get into gear and explore the second part of that principle.

The same applies if you happen to fall off the wagon. Let's say you have let your exercise regime lapse for a bit – maybe even a very long bit. Do not waste your time feeling bad about it; it happens to every-body. Just dust yourself off and get back on.

When exercise is fun and your friends or family are part of it – and when you start at a level that's right for you and keep it regular – you have the formula for success.

PART 3

Complete Health

CHAPTER 12

A Healthy Heart

Managing or reversing the effects of diabetes means more than getting your blood sugar under control. It also means regaining your health as much as you possibly can and safeguarding it.

Health problems are not a one-way street. If you have been in poor health – or if diabetes has attacked your heart, eyes, kidneys and nerves – revamping your diet can have a dramatic positive effect on your well-being. In this chapter and the next, we will look at how to keep your heart – and the rest of you – healthy.

TAKING RISK SERIOUSLY

You probably already have a good idea of your risk of heart problems. Your doctor has sized up your cholesterol level and blood pressure, and you know your family history. You may be on medications to control cholesterol or strengthen your heart.

The next step is to review what you need to know about risks, and more important, what you can do to reverse the disease process.

In evaluating your risk of developing heart problems, doctors look at your age, family history, smoking habits, weight, cholesterol level, blood pressure and other factors. I believe, however, that it is prudent to *act* as if you are at risk even if none of these factors apply to you. Here is why: most people in Europe and North America have already developed artery blockages – the beginnings of heart disease – by the time they reach early adulthood. Having diabetes increases that risk. Rather than wondering, 'Am I at risk?' it is safe to simply assume that you are – and to take action to protect yourself.

Some evidence suggests that your heart is assaulted especially hard by smoking, high blood pressure and high cholesterol levels, while your small blood vessels, such as those in your eyes and kidneys, are especially sensitive to high blood glucose levels. That is probably true, although all of these risk factors matter for both types of complications.[1,2]

SIZING UP THE ENEMY

Let's take a minute to understand the dragons we are slaying, starting with cholesterol.

Your body uses cholesterol in the same way a factory might use petroleum. Cholesterol is a raw material and your body makes many things from it. Believe it or not, cholesterol is used to make certain hormones, including testosterone and oestrogen. It is also inserted into the thin cell membranes that surround each cell in your body, and it acts as a kind of glue to hold the membranes together. Without it, you would collapse into a gelatinous heap.

Just as refineries send trucks filled with petroleum to factories to be turned into everything from plastic to petroleum jelly, your liver sends particles containing cholesterol into your bloodstream for your cells to use.

Imagine what would happen if a refinery flooded the roads with tankers, sending out far more supply than was needed. Day after day,

Is It My Genes?

Rick was 45 when he came to our office looking for help. He was not terribly optimistic that a diet change could really help him. His father had had diabetes and heart disease, and his own cholesterol had been high for years. Previous diets had let him down. A few years earlier, his doctor had suggested limiting red meat and eating more fish and chicken, but the change had had no perceptible effect. 'I've got a genetic problem,' he said. 'What I really need is a different set of parents.'

It may well be that genes played a big role in his problem, I told him. But we would not know that until we made a more serious effort to change his eating habits – one that went beyond what he had tried before.

I explained to him what you are reading in this chapter. He decided to give it a try. (His story continues on page 167.)

more and more oil trucks would clog up the roads. Some might have accidents, spilling cargo and creating havoc.

Cholesterol presents the same problem. When too many particles of cholesterol pass through your bloodstream, they create a different kind of congestion.

The circulating particles can easily become damaged. When they do, they spark the formation of raised bumps called plaques, which are very much like small scars on your artery walls.

Now, this is dangerous, because plaques are fragile. They can crack or rupture, and when that happens, the blood around the plaque starts to clot. The growing clot can fill the artery like a cork and stop blood-flow. If that happens in an artery that carries blood to the heart, a portion of heart muscle will die. That's a heart attack, which doctors call a myocardial infarction.

The solution to the problem is to reduce the number of cholesterol particles circulating in the bloodstream. Luckily, we know how to do that. Although previous diets had only a modest ability to lower cholesterol, the diet changes described within the pages of this book are dramatically effective.

REVERSING HEART DISEASE

The most famous programme using diet and lifestyle changes to tackle cholesterol and reverse heart disease was developed by Dr Dean Ornish, at the Preventive Medicine Research Institute in California.

Dr Ornish is Harvard-trained and made medical history in 1990 by showing that a combination of diet and other lifestyle changes could actually reverse artery blockages. His findings were published in the *Journal of the American Medical Association*, *Lancet* and other prestigious journals.

In his landmark study, Dr Ornish recruited heart patients from hospitals in the San Francisco area and divided them into two groups. Participants in one group – the control group – were asked to follow their regular doctors' advice about diet and other treatments. Generally speaking, that meant a diet favouring chicken and fish rather than red meat, cutting back on fat and using medications as needed.

The other group – the experimental group – was given a very different regime. They did not use cholesterol-lowering drugs at all.

Instead, they began a very special diet. First, because cholesterol is found in animal products (meat, dairy products and eggs), Dr Ornish chose a vegetarian diet for the study. Remember, grains, beans, vegetables, fruits – in fact, all plant-derived foods – are cholesterol-free.

These foods are not just free of cholesterol. They are also free of animal fat, which is even more important. Just to clarify, cholesterol and fat are two different things. Cholesterol is a microscopic ingredient in cell membranes, as described above, and is present in all animal cells.

Fat is different. It is the white strip in a cut of roast beef, the yellow layer under chicken skin and the greasy residue left on your fingers if you touch a salmon fillet. You can easily see and feel animal fat. When you eat it, your body makes cholesterol.

I learned about animal fat as a child. Some mornings, my mother cooked bacon for me and my four siblings. When it was done, she put the hot rashers on paper towels to drain. She then carefully picked up the frying pan and poured the hot grease into a jar to save it. Now, she did not store the jar of bacon grease in the refrigerator; she simply put it in the cupboard. She knew that as it cooled, it would turn into a waxy solid. The next day, she spooned some of the bacon grease into a pan and fried eggs in it. With that sort of diet, it is perhaps remarkable that any of her children lived to adulthood, but that is the way we ate until we learned better.

The fact that bacon grease is solid at room temperature is a sign that it is loaded with *saturated* fat, which you can think of as 'bad' fat, because it raises your cholesterol level.[*]

All fats are mixtures. Beef fat, for example, is about half saturated fat, with the rest being a mixture of various unsaturated fats. Chicken

---

[*] If you are wondering where the term *saturated fat* came from, it's actually very logical. If you could look at a fat molecule under a powerful microscope, it would look like a long chain of carbon atoms, with perhaps 18 or 20 atoms joined in a line. Attached to the carbon chain are hydrogen atoms. If the chain is completely covered (i.e., saturated) with hydrogen atoms, the fat becomes a waxy solid and is called a saturated fat. If, however, hydrogen atoms are absent at several spots on the fat chain, the fat is called polyunsaturated. Polyunsaturated oils are liquids. And if just one spot on the carbon chain has no hydrogen atoms attached, the fat is called monounsaturated. Olive and rapeseed oils are rich in this sort of fat. They are unusual in that they are liquid at room temperature but solid in the refrigerator. Saturated fat is the kind that pushes your cholesterol upwards.

fat is about 30 per cent saturated fat. Fish vary from about 15 to 30 per cent saturated fat. Vegetable oils are much lower in saturated fat, except for the tropical oils: coconut, palm and palm kernel oil are all high in saturated fat.

Some food companies alter vegetable oils through a process called hydrogenation, which makes them similar to saturated fats. The resulting fats, called trans fats or partially hydrogenated fats, are solid and have a long shelf life. Unfortunately, their effect on your cholesterol level is similar to that of butter or lard. They are commonly used in restaurant fryers and in snack foods. When you see the words *partially hydrogenated vegetable oil* on a food label, move along to a healthier choice.

You can see why Dr Ornish decided to use a vegetarian diet in a programme of healthy lifestyle changes. Plant foods have no cholesterol and no animal fat. He also kept vegetable oils to a minimum.

The results were remarkable. Among the vegetarians, chest pain rapidly melted away. The average person's LDL ('bad') cholesterol fell by a full 40 per cent. After a year, each participant had an angiogram − a special x-ray that shows blockages in the arteries of the heart − and Dr Ornish compared the results with those of the same kind of test done at the beginning of the study. The results were amazing: the blockages in the coronary arteries − the arteries that nourish the heart muscle itself − were actually starting to shrink. The arteries were opening again. The effect was so pronounced that the difference could be clearly seen on the angiograms of 82 per cent of patients after the first year − all with no heart bypasses, no angioplasties and not even cholesterol-lowering drugs.

WAKE UP AND SMELL THE CHOLESTEROL

By now you are probably yawning, saying you already know that cholesterol and saturated fat are bad and that we're supposed to cut down on them. 'Been there, done that,' you say.

Well, that is exactly the problem. For years, health authorities have suggested that people 'cut down' on foods containing cholesterol and animal fat. Many people have chosen leaner cuts of beef and favoured chicken and fish, but they have gotten very little in the way of results. Most people find that despite these diet changes, their cholesterol levels barely budge at all. I imagine most have decided that diet changes are a waste of time. After a month or two on their 'low-fat' diet, they find themselves ready to give up.

It turns out that a switch from red meat to white meat is not good enough. And here's why: all meats – even 'lean' meats – contain cholesterol, ranging from about 10 milligrams in every ounce of tuna to about 50 milligrams per ounce of prawns. Chicken and beef are in between, with about 25 milligrams per ounce. Red meat, poultry and fish – even the 'leaner' cuts – also contain a significant amount of fat.

In contrast, of course, there is no cholesterol or animal fat in any food from plants. That goes for every fruit and vegetable; every bean; every grain; every variety of rice, pasta and potato; and everything made from them.

Thus, if you were to try to lower your cholesterol by simply switching from beef to chicken and fish, you would have one arm tied behind your back. As shown in clinical tests, the cholesterol-lowering effect of a switch from red meat to white meat is minimal – only about 5 per cent.[3] Most people who follow such diets have no measurable improvement within their arteries, either – on average, their artery blockages continue to get worse as time goes by.

WHY DIDN'T ANYONE TELL ME?

When Dr Ornish's findings were published, most medical authorities were willing to believe his programme was a very healthy regime. But many felt the programme was so austere that few people could actually follow it. I have studied that issue in some detail, however, and have come to a completely different conclusion. The diet is not terribly austere. In fact, it stacks up well against any other diet a doctor might prescribe. Let me describe my own experience.

When I was growing up in cattle country, my family ate pretty much the same things every day: roast beef, baked potatoes and corn – except for special occasions, when we ate roast beef, baked potatoes and peas.

In medical school, I decided to change my diet. At first, I tried pasta, making a sauce from fresh tomatoes, basil and spices. Then I discovered that just below the beef, poultry and fish choices, Chinese restaurant menus feature many delicious vegetable dishes, as do Mexican restaurants. Japanese restaurants serve delicious miso soup, salads and vegetable sushi. Middle Eastern cuisine is simple but delicious, with hummus, falafel, couscous and other delights. Thai and Indian cuisines offer endless vegetarian choices. Compared to those elegant meals, my roast beef, baked potato and corn no longer seemed like the pinnacle of the culinary art. To me, a plant-based diet was a world of new tastes and was anything but austere.

When I first learned about the work of Dr Ornish in the late 1980s, I was working at the psychiatry clinic at George Washington University. I telephoned him and suggested that we study the acceptability of his diet. I flew to San Francisco and interviewed each of the participants in his heart study.[4] I asked how well they liked the foods they ate, how much effort was required to prepare them, what their family members thought and what they planned to do in the future.

I found that the vegetarian group did grumble a bit at first. They had to learn about some new foods and master some new cooking tricks. On average, it took about 4 weeks before the diet really became second nature to them. But they adapted well, partly because they saw such dramatic results. Their cholesterol levels plummeted, their chest pain disappeared and their heart disease reversed. The average participant lost, believe it or not, nearly 10 kg (22 lb) during the first year.[5,6] They came to love the foods they ate.

I vividly remember one participant's reaction. He was angry – angry that previous doctors were eager to prescribe potentially dangerous drugs and even operate on him, charging him enormous amounts of money, and did not bother to even mention the power of diet changes. Overall, the participants not only found their diets acceptable, they felt it would be wrong for doctors not to give patients this kind of choice.

Now, it did not surprise me that the vegetarian diet took a little getting used to, or that the patients soon came to love it. What surprised me was the reaction of the control group – the group that was not asked to adopt the vegetarian diet. *They* grumbled, too. Some said their diet was nothing but chicken and fish, chicken and fish, chicken and fish, night after night. All the pleasures of life were gone, some seemed to say. *And they had nothing to show for it.* Many were still dealing with chest pain, trying to control their cholesterol levels with medication and fighting a losing battle.

Having repeatedly studied how people react to different diets, I am convinced that a vegetarian diet is actually easier to follow than most other diets. This is partly because of its simplicity. Like quitting smoking or freeing yourself from any other habit, setting aside unhealthy foods is easier than teasing yourself with small amounts of them day after day. And the diet's benefits are usually so rewarding that you want to stick with it.

A few years later, I reviewed every published research study in which heart patients were asked to change their diet, with researchers tracking their success or failure.[7] At the time, the prevailing wisdom was that doctors should not push their patients too hard to make diet changes because the patients were likely to just throw up their hands and give up. But I found just the opposite. In controlled studies, when researchers asked patients to make small diet changes, they in fact achieved only small changes. When researchers encouraged their study participants to make bigger diet changes, most participants actually did make them, and they got better results. You can do it, too. Your heart deserves the very best.

AIMING TO BE HEART ATTACK–PROOF

Let's leave Dr Ornish's California research centre and take a short trip to Ohio to meet Anthony Yen. He grew up in China, where his family members routinely lived to a ripe old age. For them, heart disease, weight problems, diabetes, cancer and high blood pressure were virtually unheard of. They dined on rice, noodles and vegetable dishes of various kinds and used meat as no more than a flavouring, the way some might use bits of onion, garlic or pine nuts.

In 1949, as a young man, Anthony moved to the United States and slowly gave up his traditional Chinese diet in favour of an American one. As the years went by, he gradually gained weight, like many of his American friends, and he started to develop heart problems, which steadily worsened. Ultimately, he needed surgery – a quintuple heart bypass.

Then he was lucky enough to join a programme for heart patients run by Dr Caldwell Esselstyn Jr., aimed to get cholesterol levels so low that heart disease would stop in its tracks. He prescribed a vegetarian diet without dairy products or added oils. He showed patients how to cook and even occasionally hosted group dinners that featured home-cooked foods. He added medications only if a patient's cholesterol level did not fall below 3.8 mmol/l with diet alone.

The programme worked. Dr Esselstyn's patients became practically bulletproof. Although they were in bad shape when they arrived, no one who adhered to the programme had any sort of recurring heart problem.[8] Anthony's cholesterol level improved dramatically. He lost weight and felt better than he had in years.

In 1991 and again in 1997, Dr Esselstyn called American cardiologists together for the Summit on Cholesterol and Coronary Disease. He put forward his belief that doctors need to promote healthier diets. If doctors continue to prescribe only modestly effective diets, he said, their patients will be stuck with endless prescriptions, operating rooms will remain busy with angioplasties and coronary bypass surgeries and medical costs will continue to soar.

Dr Esselstyn was right, as Anthony Yen, his other patients, and a growing number of doctors can attest.

SPECIAL-EFFECT FOODS

By now, you know which foods to avoid. By skipping animal products and added oils, you will sidestep cholesterol and the fat that can drive cholesterol levels up. Of course, you want to avoid these foods anyway in order to improve diabetes.

There are foods you might want to *add* to your diet, though, because they can actually lower your cholesterol or protect against the damage that cholesterol can cause.

- **Oats, beans and barley** contain soluble fibre that reduces cholesterol levels. You have no doubt heard that oats, Cheerios and other oat products have this effect, and they have become popular for exactly that reason. But do not forget the cholesterol-lowering power of the humble bean, which also contains soluble fibre. Eating a 115-g (4-ounce) serving of beans every day cuts cholesterol levels significantly. People who eat beans regularly have cholesterol levels that are, on average, about 7 per cent lower than those of other people. Their LDL cholesterol is usually about 6 per cent lower, their triglycerides average 17 per cent lower and their HDL ('good') cholesterol level is about 3 per cent *higher* – all of which are good changes.[9] Soluble fibre is also found in many vegetables and fruits.

- **Soya products** have a special cholesterol-lowering effect. Aside from the fact that they have no cholesterol or animal fat, there is something about soya protein that brings down cholesterol a bit further. If your burger is made of soyabeans instead of beef, you will not only skip beef's cholesterol and fat, you will also get an extra cholesterol-lowering benefit.[10]

- **Certain nuts, such as almonds and walnuts**, lower cholesterol, too. Yes, they are as high in fat as other nuts, but somehow they have an ability to reduce cholesterol levels that has not been fully explained. In studies, eating 90 grams (3 ounces) a day for 4 weeks has shown a measurable effect.[11] I do not recommend that you make nuts a regular part of your diet, however. Despite their cholesterol-lowering effect, they are so fatty that they will make weight loss difficult and may interfere with your efforts to improve insulin sensitivity.

- **Some margarines** incorporate natural plant stanols or sterols that work almost like drugs, blocking the absorption of cholesterol from the small intestine. Benecol Light spread, for example, contains plant stanols derived from pine trees mixed into a spread made with rapeseed and soyabean oils. You can use it in baking and frying if you like. It is not a low-calorie or low-fat spread, though; 1 tablespoon has about 50 calories. Like nuts, margarines can interfere with your weight-loss efforts.

- **Garlic** may lower cholesterol, too, although not all studies are in agreement. In those that have shown an effect, the amount used was ½ to 1 clove per day.[12]

- **Fruits and vegetables** are not only cholesterol free and very low in fat; their beta-carotene, vitamin C and vitamin E can actually reduce the damaging effects of cholesterol in your blood.[13] Here's why.

    As cholesterol particles glide along in your bloodstream, those that enter artery walls and cause plaque buildup are the ones that have become slightly damaged, or oxidized. Beta-carotene, vitamin C and vitamin E actually *protect* the cholesterol particles from damage so they go on their merry way without harming you.

You will find huge amounts of beta-carotene in orange vegetables, such as carrots, sweet potatoes and pumpkins, but there is also plenty in green leafy vegetables. Vitamin C is in citrus fruits, of course, but also in many other fruits and vegetables. And whole grains, vegetables and beans are healthy sources of vitamin E.

At the University of Toronto, Dr David Jenkins took this approach to its ultimate conclusion. He reasoned that if a vegan diet (that is, one with no meat, dairy products or eggs) lowers cholesterol levels; if soluble fibre, such as that in oat bran, lowers cholesterol; if certain nuts lower cholesterol; if soya products lower cholesterol; and if plant sterols lower cholesterol, then *what would happen if he prescribed them all at the same time?*

He devised what he called a Portfolio Diet, which included all of these elements, and found that the combination led to a 29.6 per cent drop in LDL cholesterol *in just 4 weeks*, which was similar to the effect of cholesterol-lowering drugs.[14]

CONTROLLING CHOLESTEROL STEP BY STEP

Let's summarize what the research tells us about the ideal cholesterol-lowering diet. Here are the keys.

1. Skip animal products. You will want to avoid meat (that means no red meat, no chicken and no fish), dairy products and eggs. Avoid them entirely, and you will eliminate all the animal fat and cholesterol from your diet. You already know this is important for diabetes, but it is just as important for your heart.

2. Keep vegetable oils to a minimum. To trim the oil from your diet, skip the oily dressings, fried foods and foods prepared with extra oil. Read the labels on packaged foods. If you spot animal products or partially hydrogenated oils in the ingredients list, do not buy the food. And if there are more than 2 to 3 grams of fat in a serving, skip it.

3. Add special-effect foods. The best of these are oats, beans and soya products. They are filling but modest in calories and they really do bring your cholesterol down. It is easy to add special-effect foods to your routine.

Oats: Start your day with a bowl of old-fashioned oats. Top it with cinnamon if you like, but skip the milk and sugar or use soya milk.

Beans: Like oats, beans are high in soluble fibre, which lowers cholesterol. Baked beans, chickpeas, kidney beans with salsa – all are loaded with soluble fibre, protein and all-around good nutrition. The humble bean has even become quite chic, with some growers specializing in beautifully colourful heirloom varieties.

Soya: It is easy to bring soya milk into your routine. You will also want to learn about the many other forms of soya: low-fat tofu, tempeh, textured vegetable protein and many others. Some people are a bit tentative about tofu until they taste it properly prepared, then they come to love it. For all soya products, read the labels and choose those lowest in fat.

With these changes, most people can expect to see major results. Diets that eliminate cholesterol and animal fat (vegan diets), keep oils low and use special-effect foods typically achieve a 20 to 40 per cent reduction in 'bad' cholesterol.

4. If you are overweight, follow the weight-loss guidelines described in Chapter 6. Each half a kilogram or pound you lose cuts your total cholesterol by about 0.3 mmol/l.[15] The effect is gradual but important.

5. Exercise. When your doctor gives you the green light to exercise, you will find it enormously helpful. Exercise will not lower your total cholesterol, but it will increase HDL cholesterol, and that improves your overall health profile. Regular exercise (a brisk 30-minute walk five times a week or a 1-hour walk three times a week) also helps keep your blood pressure under control. Work with your doctor to set exercise goals based on your current health (see Chapter 11).

SIZING UP YOUR PROGRESS

It is easy to see if the programme is working. Follow it carefully, and after about 8 weeks, ask your doctor to check your cholesterol level. If you have not quite reached the goals you set for yourself, take a close look at what you have been eating. How well have you followed the programme? If you really did follow it carefully and your cholesterol failed to budge, you are probably one of those uncommon individuals whose genes really are driving up their cholesterol levels.

If diet alone proves insufficient, follow your doctor's advice, which

Jumping Into Oats

Rick, whom you met earlier, did very well with his diet changes despite his initial reservations. He learned how to make a quick and hearty vegetable soup from a dried soup mix to which he added tomatoes, cucumbers, sweet potatoes and whatever other vegetables he had on hand. He often cooked pasta and usually used a jar of tomato sauce for convenience. He also included plenty of salads and cooked vegetables. Eating out was a challenge for him until he discovered that ethnic restaurants had plenty of options. Speaking up helped, too – most restaurants gladly made him a vegetable option when he asked for it. He figured out which fast-food restaurants had veggie burgers or salad bars.

He took a shine to what he called fake meats – ham and other deli slices made of soya protein – which he used in sandwiches with sliced tomato, lettuce and Dijon mustard. Sometimes he had a simple meal of beans and rice or a packaged rice dish (curried rice, rice pilaf, etc.). He also became quite fond of couscous. For breakfast, he jumped into oats, figuratively speaking, and kept bananas and other fruits on hand both at home and at work.

While he found the diet surprisingly easy, he ran into a stumbling block at the beginning. He served himself modest portions and resisted going back for seconds – that felt like cheating. As a result, he often felt hungry. The fix: he simply ate more. On another occasion, he took my advice to eat beans a bit too far and had an episode of gastric distress. He cut back on his bean serving sizes for a bit and was fine.

His wife gradually adopted a vegetarian diet, too. In the process, she lost a substantial amount of weight and had more energy than she had had in years.

By the time Rick came in for his follow-up blood test, he had totally adapted to the diet, and he was thrilled with the results. In 3 months, his cholesterol had dropped from 5.2 to 3.6, with an LDL of well below 2.5. And this was the same man who had started out saying what he really needed was different genes. 'You know, this isn't a diet,' he said. 'This is a way of living, and it just feels right to me. I'm never going back to the way I used to eat. This is it.'

may include cholesterol–lowering medications. Some doctors believe that medications have value even when cholesterol levels are normal. Research is under way to test this possibility.

RAISING 'GOOD' CHOLESTEROL

The cholesterol in high-density lipoprotein (HDL) particles is called 'good' cholesterol for only one reason: it is on the way out. HDL particles scour your artery walls, picking up cholesterol and eliminating it, like tiny sanitation trucks carrying away the rubbish. If your HDL is low (see Chapter 7), the following steps will help you boost it.

1. Exercise. As you saw above, regular aerobic exercise does not have any appreciable effect on LDL cholesterol, but it can boost your HDL by about 10 per cent.[16]

2. Bring on the beans. People who eat beans or other pulses daily average a 3 per cent higher HDL value compared to that of other people.[17]

3. Eat plenty of fruits and vegetables. The vitamin C they contain appears to increase HDL, too.

4. Avoid partially hydrogenated vegetable oils. These oils do exactly the opposite of what you would like: they raise LDL cholesterol and reduce HDL. Be sure to read the fine print on labels, especially on pastries and snack foods.

5. Lose weight. A welcome side effect of a low-fat, vegan diet is weight loss, which in turn boosts HDL. The diet programme described in this book will help you.

6. If you smoke, stop. Quitting smoking boosts HDL.

REDUCING TRIGLYCERIDES

Triglycerides is a technical term for fat in the bloodstream.[*] Lowering triglycerides is a good idea, as it will probably reduce your risk of heart problems. It is usually easy to do. Take another look at the steps described above for boosting HDL, especially weight loss, exercise and introducing beans and other pulses into your menu. These steps will also cut triglycerides. Simply including beans in your daily menu is a surprisingly powerful step that trims triglycerides by as much as 17 per cent.[18] Also take one additional step: avoid sugar, white bread products

---

[*] The word *triglyceride* is derived from the fact that when your body transports fat molecules from one place to another, it generally attaches three fat molecules to a glycerine molecule (hence, *tri-glyceride*) before sending them into the watery environment of the bloodstream.

Getting the Upper Hand on Homocysteine

Homocysteine is a protein building block – an amino acid – that is normally found in small amounts in the bloodstream. If the amount in your blood is high – over 10 micromoles per litre – it may indicate an increased risk of heart problems, just as a high cholesterol level can.[19] The benefits of reducing homocysteine are not yet established, but the steps that reduce it are all healthy, so here is how to go about it.

Certain vitamins – folic acid and vitamins B_6 and B_{12} – help to eliminate homocysteine. You will find plenty of folic acid and vitamin B_6 in beans, vegetables and fruits; plant-based food sources of B_{12} are limited to supplemented products such as fortified soya milk and cereals, nutritional yeast and a few other foods.

In addition to having plenty of fruits and vegetables in your diet every day, the following is a sensible regime.

1. A multivitamin each morning. This will provide adequate folic acid, vitamin B_6 and vitamin B_{12}. Any brand is fine, but it should be free of iron since we now know that excess iron can increase the risk of heart problems.

2. A 400-microgram folic acid supplement each evening. This will boost your folic acid. If you prefer, you can take a second multivitamin that includes folic acid (see page 139).

and other high–GI foods, as discussed in Chapter 4. These foods seem to raise triglycerides, while low–GI foods that are rich in fibre seem to lower them.[20] You will probably see a big drop in your triglycerides.

ONE SOLUTION TO MANY PROBLEMS

If you have been taking all this in, you have probably come to this happy conclusion on your own: you do not need one diet for diabetes, another for cholesterol control and a third one for weight loss. A diet that skips animal products, keeps vegetable oils low and favours high-fibre, low–GI foods tackles all these problems at the same time.

Just as a drop in cholesterol is good for your heart, a drop in HbA1c is, too. People who keep their glucose under good control have fewer heart problems as the years go by.

The same diet changes also help control your blood pressure, partly because they can cause you to lose weight, and as your weight falls, so does your blood pressure. But the effect of vegetarian diets on blood pressure goes beyond their effect on weight. Plant-based diets are rich in potassium, which seems to reduce blood pressure. The absence of animal fat also reduces blood viscosity (that is, blood is less 'thick' – less like grease and more like water) so it flows more easily through the blood vessels.[21]

For many people, the effect of diet changes rivals or exceeds that of medications. If, for whatever reason, your cholesterol, blood pressure or blood sugar does not come under good control despite your best efforts, you doctor will rightly prescribe medications to take up where diet leaves off.

CHAPTER 13

Healthy Nerves, Eyes and Kidneys

Selwyn was 58 years old when he heard we were looking for volunteers for a research study. Originally from Trinidad, he had been diagnosed with diabetes almost 20 years earlier. The disease had taken a toll on his eyes, and he was being treated for glaucoma.

He also had terrible nerve pain. In the 18 months before the study began, the pain in his feet had gotten worse and worse. 'It was excruciating,' he said. 'It hurt from the calves down, especially on the left side. And it worsened as the day wore on. By the time I got home from work, I just had to put my feet up. At night, the bottoms of my feet hurt terribly, with burning and tingling.'

He had had several medical tests to search for a treatable cause, but his doctors were left with only diabetes to blame for his misery. Despite using insulin twice a day, his diabetes was not under good control.

He began doing stretching exercises, which seemed to ease the pain somewhat. When our study began, he started a low-fat, vegan diet. It suited his tastes and had a remarkable effect on his diabetes. At the beginning of the study, his HbA1c was 9.1 per cent, but his blood sugar began to fall soon after he made the switch to our eating plan. Within a month, he began to have episodes of low blood sugar, so his insulin doses were reduced. Despite the fact that he was taking less medication, his HbA1c at the 3-month point was down to 7.7. That was a big improvement, although he was not yet where he needed to be.

About 6 months into the study, something remarkable happened. 'I noticed a drastic change. I had been in total pain, but the symptoms started going away,' he said. As time went on, things got better and better. The pain became barely perceptible, and eventually – to his amazement – it disappeared altogether. 'I'm totally normal,' he said. 'I have no pain at all any more.'

If a medication could deliver the result he achieved, it would be a very popular one indeed. 'The difference has been like night and day for me,' he said.

A healthy diet does much more than keep your blood sugar down; it helps protect your whole body. If diabetes rages out of control, it can not only damage your heart, it can also attack your nerves, your eyes and your kidneys. Happily, the diet you are now beginning will help you avoid these problems. In this chapter, we will look at how to keep all your body parts in good working order.

HEALTHY NERVES

People with diabetes are at risk of nerve damage, which can take two forms.

Peripheral neuropathy, sometimes called sensorimotor neuropathy, is damage to the nerves that allow you to feel things or to move your muscles. It leads to tingling, pain, numbness or weakness in your feet or hands. It pays to take these signs seriously because although it can get better, it can also get a lot worse if you are not careful.

Reduced sensation in your feet can leave you vulnerable to injuries that you cannot feel. It is easy to overlook a small cut or scrape when you do not feel it. Injuries can also be slow to heal, which can set you up for a festering infection. Diabetes is a common cause of amputation, something that should never happen with good care.

Autonomic neuropathy is abnormalities in the nerves that control your internal functions. It can lead to digestive problems, such as nausea, vomiting, constipation or diarrhoea. It can also cause problems with bladder control or sexual function. Other symptoms include dizziness, faintness, increased or decreased sweating, visual difficulties (e.g., problems adjusting to light and dark conditions) and lack of awareness of the warning signs of low blood sugar.

The key to preventing and treating neuropathy is to get your diabetes – particularly your blood glucose level – under control, starting with diet and exercise. If neuropathy has affected you, you will want to re-read Chapter 4 and follow the diet guidelines to the letter, aiming for the best possible glucose control under the guidance of your doctor. If lifestyle changes do not do the whole job, there are medications that can help.

That said, pharmaceuticals need not be your first stop. Diet and exercise can be surprisingly powerful. At California's Weimar Institute of Health and Education, Dr Milton Crane asked 21 diabetes patients with peripheral neuropathy to do two things: begin a low-fat, vegan diet and take a daily 30-minute walk. The effects were rapid and very strong: within 2 weeks, leg pains stopped completely in 17 of the participants and the remaining 4 had partial relief.[1]

Supplements for Treating Neuropathy

Researchers have tested the effects of the following supplements, all of which are subjects of further research to determine whether they work, in what dosages, and for whom. The verdicts are not yet in on them as treatments for nerve damage, so I'm listing them here not as a recommendation but simply to make you aware of them.

Alpha-lipoic acid appears to improve neuropathy symptoms.[2] It is a strong antioxidant and may also improve circulation. Studies have used both intravenous and oral doses, but optimal dosages are not yet established.

Gamma-linolenic acid is an omega-6 fatty acid commonly sold in health food stores. At doses of 480 milligrams per day, it appears to reduce neuropathy symptoms.[3]

Carnitine, in doses of 1,000 milligrams daily, reduced pain in patients with diabetic neuropathy.[4]

Magnesium supplements, in doses of 300 milligrams per day, appear to slow the progression of neuropathy over the long term.[5]

If You Have Nerve Damage

If the nerves of your feet have been damaged, it is important that you get regular checkups and protect your feet. If you have lost some feeling, check your feet daily for any sign of injury or infection, such as redness or swelling, and have it treated right away. Avoid walking barefoot. If you have lost some feeling in your feet, you may not know if you step on something that breaks the skin. Be sure your shoes fit properly to avoid blisters and break in new shoes slowly. Keep your nails in good shape and do not trim them shorter than the ends of your toes. If your vision is poor or you have difficulty safely trimming your nails, have a podiatrist examine your feet and trim your nails.

HEALTHY EYES

Your eyes are delicate cameras that capture the world around you, transmitting its details to your brain to perceive and remember. In the same way that a camera is fragile, several parts of the eye are susceptible to damage. This is true for anyone, but especially for people with diabetes. Protecting your eyes means keeping your blood glucose, blood pressure and cholesterol under control.

Three parts of the eye are particularly vulnerable. First, pressure can build up in the front part of the eye – called the anterior chamber – and eventually damage the retina and optic nerve. This is a condition called glaucoma. Second, a cataract can compromise the lens's clarity. Third, blood vessels in the retina can become damaged. Let's look at what we can do to prevent this three-pronged assault.

Glaucoma

There are several different types of glaucoma. Typically, increasing pressure within the eye pinches the tiny blood vessels in the retina, damaging it and the optic nerve. High blood pressure and high glucose levels both increase your risk of developing glaucoma. Your best defence is to get both under control, using the information in this chapter and the rest of this book. If glaucoma is caught early, treatment (with prescription eyedrops) is highly effective.

Glaucoma can begin with no symptoms at all, so it is important to have eye examinations by an ophthalmic optometrist at least once a year.

Cataracts

If the lens of the eye loses its clarity, becoming more like waxed paper than like a crystalline pane of glass, a doctor diagnoses a cataract. You may experience blurred or double vision, difficulty with distance vision, a halo effect around lights, or excessive glare in bright sunlight or while driving at night.

While cataract surgery has advanced dramatically in recent years, the ideal situation is to keep your original equipment in good working order. Luckily, there are several things you can do to help prevent cataracts.

First, it is important to avoid tobacco and to protect your eyes from harsh sunlight.

Second, it pays to follow the same diet steps that apply to controlling diabetes in general, as described in Chapter 4. That means avoiding animal products, keeping oils to a minimum and favouring low-GI foods. There is evidence that these steps reduce your risk – specifically, people who avoid fatty foods tend to have less cataract risk.[6]

The same appears to be true for people who avoid dairy products. Generally speaking, people who steer clear of dairy products appear to have significantly less risk of developing cataracts.[7] The culprit here appears to be lactose, or milk sugar, rather than milk fat.

During the digestive process, lactose releases a simple sugar called galactose, which can enter the lens. Infants who lack the enzymes necessary to break down galactose develop cataracts within the first year of life. The relationship between dairy products and cataracts is still being studied, but this is one more good reason to avoid them.

Certain foods help protect the eyes. Particularly valuable are green leafy vegetables such as broccoli, spinach, kale and mustard greens. These are rich sources of certain antioxidants, called lutein[8] and zeaxanthin, which protect the lens.[9] Foods rich in vitamins C and E may help, too.[10] You will find plenty of vitamin C in oranges, peppers, cantaloupe melon, strawberries and kiwifruit. It also shows up in places you may not expect: cruciferous vegetables – broccoli, brussels sprouts, cauliflower and kale – as well as tomatoes and sweet potatoes. Healthy sources of vitamin E include cooked spinach, soya milk, mangoes, wheat germ, and, of course, most multivitamins.

Finally, people who avoid alcohol have about 10 per cent less cataract risk than other people. Even very modest consumption, about two drinks per week, is linked to increased risk.[11]

Retinopathy

The retina, located at the back of your eye, is like camera film. Millions of tiny nerves in the retina pick up images and send them to the brain. Also like film, your retinas are fragile. They can be damaged by elevated blood glucose, blood pressure or cholesterol, leading to a condition called retinopathy, meaning damage to the retina. The condition occurs in two main forms.

Non-proliferative retinopathy occurs when capillaries balloon out and leak substances into the retina, leading to the formation of fatty deposits. In most cases, the condition is mild and needs no treatment, but it is essential that an ophthalmologist checks your eyes regularly to be sure the condition does not become more serious.

Proliferative retinopathy occurs when blood vessels are so damaged that they begin to close off. When that happens, new, abnormal vessels start to form in the retina. The new vessels are fragile and prone to bleeding, leading to scarring and sometimes even to retinal detachment. Ophthalmologists use laser treatments to treat the abnormal vessels.

Most people with diabetes eventually develop at least a mild degree of retinopathy. The good news is that there is a lot you can do to prevent serious problems. Good blood glucose control protects the eyes,[12] and by now you know how to go about attaining that. Keeping blood pressure[13] and cholesterol[14] down helps, too. The diet steps above will

The Eye

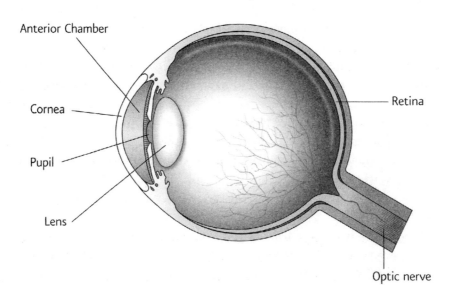

go a long way towards helping you reach that goal. If diet alone is insufficient, your doctor will add medications as needed.

Retinopathy begins without symptoms, so it is essential to have your eyes checked regularly and to choose your foods as if your vision depended on it. It does.

HEALTHY KIDNEYS

Your kidneys are made up of millions of tiny filtration units. They purify your blood, sending waste products out into the urine and holding on to proteins and other normal blood components. But just as the retina's tiny blood vessels can be damaged, so can these tiny vessels in your kidneys. High blood pressure, high blood glucose and high cholesterol assault them, leading to a condition doctors call nephropathy.

Left uncontrolled, kidney damage can progress to the point where your options boil down to dialysis or kidney transplant. Needless to say, you do not want anything like that to happen. Here are the diet steps you need to take.

First, follow the basic diet guidelines for diabetes as described in Chapter 4. The need is not just for avoiding fat and cholesterol and keeping your blood glucose and cholesterol down, although those are very important.[15] Animal protein is part of the problem, too, so you want to avoid it. Since animal protein taxes the kidneys, getting your protein from plant sources helps protect them.[16–18]

This is an important point, so stick with me while I explain: many people imagine that egg white, chicken breast or haddock are healthy foods because they are high in protein – but that very fact is what makes them undesirable. The less animal protein you consume, the lower your risk of kidney problems. You are much safer getting your protein from plant sources – beans, vegetables and grains, for example.

A low-fat, vegan diet is not only free of animal protein, cholesterol and animal fat, it also helps bring down high blood pressure,[19] which is also important for protecting your kidneys.

It goes without saying that you should avoid tobacco. Among its many ill effects, smoking damages blood vessels.

If your blood pressure, glucose or cholesterol remain high despite your best efforts, your doctor will prescribe medications to bring them under control. Some doctors prescribe medications even if your tests are in the normal range, as a means of protecting kidney tissues. This is done on an individualized basis.

In our recent study, we tracked the kidney health of our participants. They dutifully collected their urine twice over two 24-hour periods so we could measure their albumin losses (your doctor will probably use less arduous tests). They did this before beginning their assigned new diets and again after following them for 22 weeks.

During this time, the group following the American Diabetes Association diet had a 21 per cent average drop in albumin losses. That's a change in the right direction. However, the vegan group had the advantage of consuming no animal protein, animal fat or cholesterol, and its average albumin losses were 56 per cent, falling to less than half of their beginning values.

GETTING HEALTHY AND STAYING THAT WAY

If you have been gaining weight, needing more and more medications, or developing one or many complications, my goal is to help you change course. We now know that it is possible to lose weight effectively and permanently, reduce or eliminate medications, reverse heart disease and even improve the symptoms of neuropathy. If you thought you had to surrender to advancing symptoms, think again. You are now in the driver's seat.

CHAPTER 14

Information for Doctors and Diabetes Nurses

Although this book is intended as a tool for people with diabetes, there are a few key points I would like to mention to doctors and other heath care providers. As you will see, this programme is both very effective and highly engaging. While health care providers are used to seeing their patients becoming frustrated with typical 'diabetes diets' and requiring ever-higher medication dosages, both doctors and patients find this approach fresh and rewarding.

Health care providers play key roles for individuals on this programme, just as they do with any diabetes treatment programme. They educate and encourage their patients, and monitor their progress.

In the research studies we have conducted, we have found that many patients treated with insulin or insulin secretogogues have hypoglycaemic episodes as they improve their diets. As your patients embark on this new diet, you will need to prepare them for that possibility and be ready to reduce their medications as needed. It is also important that they understand that the hypoglycaemia was caused by the medications, not by any defect in their physiology. More on this below.

THE ROLE OF THE HEALTH CARE PROVIDER

There are many ways doctors and other health care providers can help patients as they begin major dietary changes. First, of course, is encouragement. Many patients have seen their parents or grandparents end up with frightening diabetes complications, such as eye problems, loss of kidney function or amputations, and many have already begun to experience neuropathy or other problems by the time they decide to take the disease seriously. They need to know that they can avoid these problems – as indeed they can – if they follow your advice, including maintaining a good diet.

It is helpful for them to know that this is not the same diabetes diet they may have already tried and that they will need to learn a few new tricks. They will discover new products, new restaurants and perhaps new menu items at their favourite restaurants. The most helpful doctors learn about these diet choices, too. If you have not yet tried a low-fat, vegan diet, I would strongly encourage you to do so. Apart from its health benefits, the experience will also prepare you to answer patients' questions and offer encouragement.

One way to help patients get started on this programme is to identify a limited period – say, 3 weeks – in which to give the diet a good try. For now, there is no need to commit to it forever, but during this short period, they would do well to follow it 100 per cent so they can experience its full effect. Once they see how it works, they will probably want to continue.

Avoid the temptation to water down the diet. Doctors who tell patients to follow a diet 'most of the time' or to 'just do the best you can' tacitly encourage them to deviate from it. We never do that when patients have alcohol or tobacco problems, because we know that it is easier to stick to a consistent programme than to try to negotiate with these problem substances. The same is true of food; it is better to encourage patients to give it 100 per cent, never setting a foot wrong.

Occasionally, some patients will slip back into their old diet habits. When that happens, they will almost instantly notice that they no longer manage their weight as well, and their blood glucose levels will start to climb again. They will also arrive at your surgery with a heavy burden of guilt. Many will speak of foods as 'sinful', 'decadent', 'naughty', etc. I suggest that you remain positive, avoid moralizing and return the focus to biology, which is where it belongs. Patients who have returned fat to their diets may well be packing their cells with more intramyocellular lipid, which is likely to harm their insulin sensitivity. Encourage them to dust themselves off and get back on the wagon.

Some patients need to be encouraged to eat carbohydrate-rich foods. Because of the carbohydrate counting they have already learned, they may have come to see all carbohydrates as unhealthy. This feeling was aided and abetted by the low-carbohydrate diet craze. It is important to remind patients that countries whose populations have traditionally consumed high-carbohydrate diets – such as Asian countries, where rice and noodles are dietary staples and meat and dairy consumption is much less prevalent than in Western countries – have historically had very low diabetes rates.

You can also help patients ensure nutritional adequacy by asking them to take a daily multivitamin. This is good advice for all patients, of course, but to get adequate vitamin B_{12}, it is much easier to take a daily multivitamin than to try to remember which vegan foods are B_{12}-enriched.

HYPOGLYCAEMIA

Patients who are taking insulin or insulin secretogogues are subject to hypoglycaemia. If they improve their diets and begin to lose weight, hypoglycaemic episodes are common. In my experience, most patients on insulin and about half of all patients on a sulfonylurea or nateglinide who begin a low-fat, vegan diet have hypoglycaemic episodes, usually within the first several weeks.

Patients will be delighted to know that they have improved so much that their medications are now too strong, but they will also be concerned about what hypoglycaemia means. It is important for them to understand that it was caused by their medication and that it does not indicate that there is anything wrong with them. It is also essential for them to know, right from the outset, what to do and whom to call when these episodes happen. Of course, the initial steps – checking their blood glucose and taking glucose tablets or food – are things they can do on their own. But it is important to provide specific instructions and to ask patients to carry your telephone number (or that of an office backup) with them and use it as necessary – even on weekends – so you can adjust their medications. You will find my instructions for patients on dealing with hypoglycaemia beginning on page 98.

Menus and Recipes

The following menus and recipes were developed and tested by Bryanna Clark Grogan, a chef, recipe developer and food writer. Her many cookbooks cover an enormous range of foods and cooking styles, from quick and easy recipes to many kinds of ethnic cuisine.

Bryanna's recipes are full-bodied, savoury dishes with a special 'something'. You will notice that their flavours go beyond the tastes and aromas of the individual ingredients. The blends of simple foods and well-chosen spices make each recipe special.

It may be that she is tapping into the so-called fifth flavour. While Western palates expect the usual sweet, salty, sour and bitter tastes, culinary scientists discovered long ago that the tongue perceives a fifth flavour that might best be called a *savoury* taste (Asian cooks call it *umami*). For decades, food researchers have investigated how this flavour response is triggered by meaty dishes and accentuated by flavour enhancers, such as monosodium glutamate. Health-conscious cooks, of course, prefer to release flavours with healthy ingredients. As Bryanna has found, certain food combinations do indeed accentuate savoury flavours and aromas.

This recipe collection is intended for a wide range of tastes and temperaments and includes both simple and more adventurous offerings. When we have included an unusual ingredient, you can find more information in Appendix 2. Thanks to Gabrielle Turner-McGrievy and Jennifer Reilly who contributed additional recipes.

HOW TO STEAM-FRY

Some recipes call for steam-frying, a technique for sautéing or stir-frying without fat. Here is how to do it.

Place a heavy nonstick frying pan over medium heat and add the ingredients to be cooked (e.g., chopped onions or other vegetables). Then add 1 to 2 tablespoons of liquid (water, low-sodium vegetable stock or wine) – just enough to keep the food from sticking. Do not crowd the pan, or the vegetables will stew.

Increase the heat to high and cook until the liquid starts to evaporate, stirring with a wooden spatula or spoon until the vegetables are done to your liking.

You can brown onions perfectly by this method. As soon as the natural sugars in the onions start to brown on the bottom and edges of the pan, add a little more liquid and mix the browned portions with the remaining onions. Continue until the onions are soft and brown, being careful not to scorch them.

To steam-fry in a microwave, use a glass dish, such as a round 25-cm (10-in) glass baking dish. Add the ingredients, including the 1 to 2 tablespoons of liquid, and cover with a glass lid or microwaveable plate. Microwave on high for 5 minutes or until the vegetables are soft, then add to the recipe. As almost everyone with a microwave knows, you can cook vegetables in it, but you cannot brown them or any other food. If you like a brown, crispy texture, stick with the stovetop method.

7 Days of Healthy Meals

DAY 1

Breakfast

Oats cooked with apples

Soya milk

Lunch

Black-Eyed Bean and Sweet Potato Soup (page 210)

Toasted rye or sprouted-grain bread

Spinach salad with mandarin orange segments and *Creamy Poppy Seed Dressing* (page 205)

Snack

Fruit Smoothie (page 195)

Dinner

Lebanese-Style Lentils and Pasta (page 226)

Steamed broccoli

Orange and Apple Date Cake (page 241)

DAY 2

Breakfast

Wheatberry pancakes (page 197)

Sliced berries

Soya yogurt

Lunch

Spinach Hummus (page 200) and vegetables of choice wrapped in a wholewheat tortilla

Orange Quinoa and Bulgur Tabbouleh (page 216)

Snack

Baked corn chips, salsa and *Vegetarian 'Refried' Beans* (page 199)

Dinner

Indonesian-Style Stir-Fried Pasta (page 230)

Thai-Style Coleslaw (page 216)

Fresh fruit

DAY 3

Breakfast

Tofu Scramblers (page 192)

Rye toast

Fruit salad

Lunch

Panini sandwich made with sprouted-grain bread, *Tofu Mayonnaise* (page 222), low-fat vegetarian 'meat' slices and rocket

Creamy Mushroom Soup (page 208)

Snack

Apple slices dipped in *Lemon Crème* (page 242)

Dinner

Lemon and Artichoke Tagine (page 227)

Orange Couscous Pilaf (page 234)

Baby mixed greens salad with *Creamy Black Pepper Dressing* (page 206)

Berry Mousse (page 244)

DAY 4

Breakfast

Breakfast Barley with Fruit (page 191)

Soya milk

Lunch

Red Lentil and Sweet Potato Soup (page 211)

Italian Stuffed Griddle Dumplings (page 214)

Snack

Raw vegetables

Wholegrain rye-crisp crackers

Spinach Hummus (page 200)

Dinner

Aubergine Parmesan (page 232)

Green salad with *Balsamic Vinaigrette* (page 203)

Bulgur Wheat and Quinoa Pilaf (page 236)

Fresh fruit

DAY 5

Breakfast

Toasted sprouted-grain bread

Low-fat vegetarian sausage

Grilled mushrooms and tomato

Lunch

Black Bean Soft Tacos (page 212)

Cherry Tomato and Brown Rice Salad with Artichoke Hearts (page 218)

Snack

Orange and Apple Date Cake (page 241)

Non-dairy milk

Dinner

Savoury Soya Roast (page 223)

Crusty rye bread

Brussels Sprouts with Lemon and Vegetarian Bacon (page 235)

Fresh fruit

DAY 6

Breakfast

Muesli Cereal (page 193)

Soya milk

Fresh fruit

Lunch

Mediterranean Veggie Panini (page 215)

Sautéed Portabella Mushroom Salad (page 221)

Snack

Wholegrain crackers

Cypriot Yellow Split Pea and Dill Spread (page 201)

Dinner

White Bean and Sweet Potato Stew (page 225)

Sprouted-grain bread

Steamed broccoli and courgettes

Gingerbread Cake (page 240) with *Lemon Crème* (page 242)

DAY 7

Breakfast

Breakfast Burgers (page 196)

Tofu Scramblers (page 192)

Lunch

Barley and Winter Squash Soup (page 208)

Oatmeal Drop Scones (page 194)

Red Cabbage Slaw with Cranberries and Apples (page 220)

Snack

Pineapple Lolly Pops (page 243)

Dinner

Vegetarian Mixed-Bean Chilli (page 229)

Rye bread

BLT Salad (page 222)

Crispy Fruit Chimichangas (page 242)

Breakfasts

Breakfast Barley with Fruit

For delicious taste, lots of soluble fibre and a wonderfully low gly-caemic index, try barley flakes for your breakfast porridge. It takes a bit longer to cook than oats unless you soak it the night before. Serve with your favourite non-dairy milk and a touch of brown sugar or the sweetener of your choice.

30 g (1 oz) rolled barley (barley flakes)
⅛ teaspoon salt
180 ml (6 fl oz) water
1 tablespoon wheat bran
½ medium apple with peel, cored and chopped, or other
    chopped fruit
1½ teaspoons ground flaxseed

The night before: Combine the barley, salt and water in a microwave-able bowl, cover and refrigerate overnight. (Be sure to use a large bowl – barley can really boil up!)

In the morning: Add the bran and apple or other fruit to the soaked barley. Cover the bowl with a microwaveable plate and microwave on high for 2 minutes. Finish cooking on medium for 4 minutes. Stir in the flaxseed.

To cook on the hob: Bring the soaked barley, bran and apple or other fruit to the boil in a small nonstick saucepan over high heat, stirring. Reduce the heat to low, partially cover, and simmer for about 15 minutes, stirring occasionally. The mixture should have the consistency of cooked oats. If it's too watery, continue cooking over low heat to desired consistency.

MAKES 1 SERVING

Per serving: 197 calories/825 kJ, 6 g protein, 8 g carbohydrates, 8 g sugar, 2 g total fat, 10% calories from fat, 42 g fibre, 252 mg sodium

Tofu Scramblers

It takes about the same amount of time to make Tofu Scramblers as it does to make scrambled eggs when you use the handy homemade mix. Shake or stir the mix before measuring. Onion powder is a great store cupboard item as it's so convenient to use. It isn't as widely available as it used to be but you can get good quality organic onion powder on the Internet.

Scrambler Mix
30 g (1 oz) nutritional yeast flakes
5 tablespoons + 1 teaspoon onion powder
4 teaspoons curry powder
4 teaspoons salt
4 teaspoons ground turmeric
4 teaspoons ground cumin

Scramblers
1½ teaspoons Tofu Scrambler Mix
115 g (4 oz) reduced-fat extra-firm silken tofu, crumbled
2 tablespoons reduced-fat soya milk (optional)

For the mix: Blend the yeast flakes, onion powder, curry powder, salt, turmeric and cumin in a dry blender or mini-processor. Store in a covered jar.

For the scramblers: Combine the scrambler mix and tofu well in a medium bowl. Add the soya milk, if desired. Cook the mixture in a heavy nonstick frying pan until it reaches the desired consistency, stirring constantly with a plastic spatula or wooden spoon.

To microwave, combine the ingredients in a microwaveable dish, cover and cook on high (for 115 g/4 oz, about 2 minutes; for 230 g/8 oz, about 3½ minutes; for 340 g/12 oz, about 5 minutes; and for 455 g/16 oz, about 7½ minutes).

MAKES 1 SERVING

Per serving: 54 calories/226 kJ, 9 g protein, 3 g carbohydrates, 1 g sugar, 1 g total fat, 15% calories from fat, 1 g fibre, 252 mg sodium

Variations

If you like, add chopped vegetarian bacon or ham; steam-fried chopped onions, spring onions, mushrooms, peppers or tomatoes. If cooking in the microwave, place the vegetables in the bottom of the dish, put the tofu (mixed with the scrambler mix) on top and cook as usual, then stir together before serving.

Muesli Cereal

Bircher muesli was invented in Switzerland as a nutritious raw but digestible breakfast cereal. You can buy expensive commercial versions, but the original is low in fat, easy to make and quick, as long as you remember to start the night before. Serve muesli with reduced-fat non-dairy milk or soya yogurt; brown sugar, maple syrup or agave syrup to taste; and fresh fruit (such as berries), if desired.

125 g (4½ oz) rolled oats or other rolled wholegrain cereal
350 ml (12 fl oz) water
2 tablespoons wheat bran
2 tablespoons currants, raisins or other dried fruit
¼ teaspoon salt
2 medium apples with peel, grated
3 tablespoons lemon juice

The night before: Combine the oats and water in a bowl and refrigerate overnight.

Just before serving: Add the bran, currants or raisins, salt, apples and lemon juice to the soaked oats.

Note: To make 1 serving, use 6 tablespoons oats; 6 tablespoons water; 1 teaspoon bran; 1 teaspoon dried fruit; a pinch of salt; ½ small apple, grated; and 2¼ teaspoons lemon juice.

MAKES 4 SERVINGS

Per serving: 173 calories/724 kJ, 6 g protein, 36 g carbohydrates, 11 g sugar, 2 g total fat, 10% calories from fat, 6 g fibre, 122 mg sodium

Oatmeal Drop Scones

Traditional Scottish *skon* recipes contained no fat at all. They were eaten immediately, warm and fresh, as these should be. Enjoy them with low-sugar jam.

90 g (3 oz) old-fashioned oats
150 g (5½ oz) wholemeal flour
1 teaspoon sugar
½ teaspoon bicarbonate of soda
½ teaspoon salt
300 ml (10 fl oz) reduced-fat soya milk
1 tablespoon lemon juice or vinegar
Sugar or caraway seed

Preheat the oven to 200°C/400°F/gas 6. Grind the oats to a fine meal in a food processor. Pour into a medium bowl and add the flour, sugar, bicarbonate of soda and salt. Mix well.

Mix the soya milk and lemon juice or vinegar in a small bowl. Pour into the dry mixture and stir briefly with a fork. Drop by large spoonfuls onto 2 nonstick baking sheets (or baking sheets lined with parchment), making 12 mounds. Smooth the tops a bit with wet fingertips. Bake for about 15 minutes. Split with a fork while still hot.

For a bannock shape: divide the dough in half, and with wet hands, pat the dough pieces into 20 cm (8 in) circles in two 23 cm (9 in) nonstick cake tins (or cake tins lined with parchment cut to fit). Score each circle into 6 wedges and bake for 15 to 20 minutes.

Sprinkle with the sugar or caraway seed.

MAKES 12 SERVINGS

Per serving: 77 calories/322 kJ, 3 g protein, 15 g carbohydrates, 1 g sugar, 1 g total fat, 9% calories from fat, 2 g fibre, 144 mg sodium

Variations
Currant Scones: Add 30–60 g (1–2 oz) dried currants. You can also add 1 grated apple.
Herb Scones: Add 3 tablespoons loosely packed chopped fresh herbs of your choice.

Herb Bannock: This resembles a focaccia, is quick to make and is a great snack. Add 3 tablespoons fresh herbs to the oatmeal scone dough. Divide the dough in half and follow the instructions for making the bannock shape. Make indentations all over the dough with your fingertips. Spray the tops lightly with water from a mist sprayer and sprinkle with coarse salt or soya Parmesan, or top with steam-fried or grilled chopped mushrooms, garlic, peppers and/or onions. Serve with balsamic vinegar for dipping.

Fruit Smoothie

This quick and easy recipe is great way to start your day – or give you a healthy boost anytime.

120 ml (4 fl oz) unsweetened apple or orange juice
120 ml (4 fl oz) reduced-fat soya milk
75 g (2½ oz) frozen blueberries or other berries
75 g (2½ oz) frozen or fresh peach slices
1 tablespoon soya protein powder

Combine the juice, soya milk, berries, peaches and protein powder in a blender or food processor. Blend until very smooth.

MAKES 1 SERVING

Per serving: 148 calories/620 kJ, 4 g protein, 32 g carbohydrates, 13 g sugar, 2 g total fat, 9% calories from fat, 3 g fibre, 65 mg sodium

Breakfast Burgers

These burgers make a great breakfast on their own or alongside Tofu Scramblers (page 192). Serve them with ketchup or apple sauce.

2 large onions, finely chopped
340 g (12 oz) dried, cooked (or tinned) pinto beans or kidney
   beans, rinsed and drained
150 g (5½ oz) quick-cooking oats or porridge oats
30 g (1 oz) chickpea flour (besan) or low-fat soya flour
6 tablespoons hot water
1 tablespoon low-sodium soy sauce
1 teaspoon salt
½ teaspoon dried thyme
½ teaspoon dried sage
½ teaspoon garlic granules

In a large, heavy nonstick frying pan, steam-fry the onions over high heat until softened, adding drops of water as needed to keep them from sticking. Or cook covered in a microwave at high power for 3 to 5 minutes.

Mash the beans coarsely on a plate with a fork.

In a medium bowl, mix the mashed beans, oats, chickpea or soy a flour, hot water, soy sauce, salt, thyme, sage and garlic granules. Add the onions and mix well. At this point, you can cover the bowl and refrigerate the mixture for up to three days.

When ready to cook, form the mixture into 20 thin burgers, placing them on a baking sheet lined with baking parchment. Cook the burgers a few at a time on a heavy nonstick frying pan over medium-low heat for about 3 minutes per side, covering the pan. They should be well-browned and slightly crispy. Serve hot.

MAKES 5 (4 BURGER) SERVINGS

YIELD: 20 BURGERS

Per serving: 254 calories/1063 kJ, 13 g protein, 46 g carbohydrates, 3 g sugar, 3 g total fat, 8% calories from fat, 11 g fibre, 505 mg sodium

Wheatberry Pancakes

Who would guess that with the help of your blender, you could make deliciously light pancakes from freshly ground wheat in minutes? Try these!

150 g (5½ oz) wheat berries (wholewheat kernels)
1 tablespoon whole flaxseed
480 ml (16 fl oz) water
30 g (1 oz) chickpea flour (besan) or low-fat soya flour
1 tablespoon sugar
2 teaspoons lemon juice
2 teaspoons baking powder
½ teaspoon bicarbonate of soda
½ teaspoon salt

Place the wheat berries, flaxseed and water in a blender and process at high speed for about 2 minutes. Add the flour and process for 2 to 3 minutes or until very smooth. Add the sugar, lemon juice, baking powder, bicarbonate of soda and salt and process until well mixed.

Heat a heavy nonstick griddle or frying pan over high heat until drops of water dance on the surface and then quickly disappear. Reduce the heat to medium-high. Working in batches if necessary, pour dollops of batter quickly onto the griddle, leaving space to expand. When bubbles appear on the surface, gently flip the pancakes. Don't overcook; they should be a bit puffy when you take them off the griddle, so they are light and cakey.

MAKES 12 X 10 cm (4 in) PANCAKES (3 SERVINGS)

Per serving: 261 calories/1093 kJ, 11 g protein, 53 g carbohydrates, 6 g sugar, 3 g total fat, 9% calories from fat, 9 g fibre, 534 mg sodium

Dips, Spreads and Dressings

Low-Fat Guacamole

This 'mock-amole' is creamy and tasty. It is delicious with baked corn tortilla chips.

145 g (5 oz) fresh green beans or frozen small whole green beans
145 g (5 oz) butter beans
90 g (3 oz) reduced-fat firm or extra-firm silken tofu
3 tablespoons lemon juice
2 cloves garlic, crushed
¾ teaspoon salt
½ teaspoon ground cumin
4 tablespoons chunky no-sugar-added tomato salsa

Cook the green beans in enough water to cover for about 5 minutes or just until tender but not mushy. Drain well, transfer to a food processor, add the butter beans and blend until smooth.

Add the tofu, lemon juice, garlic, salt and cumin and blend until smooth. Add the salsa and pulse briefly to mix. Scoop into a covered bowl and refrigerate.

MAKES ABOUT 8 SERVINGS

Per 60 ml (2 fl oz) serving: 37 calories/155 kJ, 2 g protein, 7 g carbohydrates, 1 g sugar, 0.5 g total fat, 5% calories from fat, 2 g fibre, 226 mg sodium

Vegetarian 'Refried' Beans

This fat-free version of refried beans has a light texture and can be made with a variety of beans. It also makes a great warm bean dip or a delicious cold spread for sandwiches, wraps or crackers.

3 × 420 g tins black, kidney or pinto beans, rinsed and drained
1 small onion, finely chopped
2 tablespoons red wine vinegar
1 teaspoon salt
1 teaspoon ground cumin
1 teaspoon dried oregano
1 teaspoon dried garlic granules
1 teaspoon chilli powder
Hot pepper sauce to taste (optional)

Place the beans, onion, vinegar, salt, cumin, oregano, garlic granules, chilli powder and hot pepper sauce, if desired, in a food processor. Blend for several minutes or until very smooth. Transfer to a serving bowl, cover and refrigerate.

For a hot dip, microwave on high for about 3 minutes or heat in a frying pan, stirring constantly.

MAKES ABOUT 16 SERVINGS

Per 60 ml (2 fl oz) serving: 68 calories/285 kJ, 4 g protein, 12 g carbohydrates, 0.5 g sugar, 0.5 g total fat, 4% calories from fat, 4 g fibre, 120 mg sodium

Spinach Hummus

Most versions of this popular Middle Eastern chickpea dip are chock-full of olive oil and sesame tahini. This recipe contains a little tahini and plenty of spinach or other greens for good nutrition and lots of colour. Serve with raw veggies and dark rye-crisp crackers. Heating the chickpeas before processing makes a creamier hummus.

285 g (10 oz) frozen spinach, thawed
340 g (12 oz) well-cooked chickpeas
80 ml (3 fl oz) lemon juice
1 tablespoon sesame tahini
4–6 cloves garlic
1½ teaspoons salt
1 teaspoon ground cumin
¼ teaspoon cayenne pepper

Squeeze as much liquid from the spinach as you can and chop with a sharp knife. Set aside.

Place the chickpeas, lemon juice, tahini, garlic, salt, cumin and cayenne in a food processor. Blend until as smooth as desired, adding a bit of water if necessary (it will thicken somewhat in the refrigerator). Add the spinach and blend briefly.

Transfer to a serving bowl, cover with clingfilm and refrigerate until ready to serve.

MAKES ABOUT 12 SERVINGS

Per 60 ml (2 fl oz) serving: 107 calories/448 kJ, 7 g protein, 19 g carbohydrates, 0.5 g sugar, 2 g total fat, 13% calories from fat, 6 g fibre, 336 mg sodium

Variations
For a more traditional hummus, omit the greens and decrease the salt to 1 teaspoon, the cumin to ½ teaspoon and the cayenne to a pinch.
For delicious red pepper hummus, make the traditional hummus variation and add 4 large pieces drained and rinsed roasted red peppers from a jar when you process the chickpeas.

Cypriot Yellow Split Pea and Dill Spread

This easy spread is delicious with dark rye-crisp crackers. The garlic mellows considerably when cooked.

230 g (8 oz) dried yellow split peas
7 cloves garlic
1 small onion, chopped
1 teaspoon salt
700 ml (1¼ pt) water
3 tablespoons fresh lemon juice
2 teaspoons dried dill weed or 2 tablespoons chopped fresh dill
Freshly ground black pepper to taste
Paprika (optional)
1 sprig fresh dill (optional)

Combine the split peas, 6 of the garlic cloves, onion, salt and water in a medium saucepan. Bring to the boil, skimming off any foam. Reduce the heat, cover and simmer for 30 minutes.

Transfer to a food processor or blender and process, or use a hand-held blender in the pan. (Remove the 'pusher' from the top of the food processor so hot air can escape. Cover the hole loosely with a folded clean cloth while processing.) Crush the remaining garlic clove and add to the mixture along with the lemon juice and dill. Process until very smooth. Season with the pepper.

Pour into a decorative serving bowl, cover and let cool. Garnish with the paprika and dill sprig, if desired.

This spread is best served at room temperature. If you store it in the refrigerator, simply bring it to room temperature before serving.

MAKES ABOUT 10 SERVINGS

Per 60 ml (2 fl oz) serving: 74 calories/310 kJ, 5 g protein, 14 g carbohydrates, 2 g sugar, 0.5 g total fat, 2% calories from fat, 5 g fibre, 193 mg sodium

White Bean and Sun-Dried Tomato Spread

This chunky dip or spread can be served warm or at room temperature with dark rye crispbreads, sprouted bread or raw vegetables. It also makes a great spread for wraps.

20 g (¾ oz) sun-dried tomatoes (not packed in oil), chopped
1 large onion, finely chopped
2 cloves garlic, crushed
120 ml (4 fl oz) low-sodium vegetarian stock
420 g tin cannellini or other white beans
1½ tablespoons white wine vinegar or fresh lemon juice
2 tablespoons finely chopped parsley
½ teaspoon salt
¼ teaspoon dried thyme
¼ teaspoon dried marjoram or basil
White pepper to taste

In a small bowl, cover the sun-dried tomatoes with 120 ml (4 fl oz) boiling water. Let them soak, covered, for 10 minutes, or until softened. Drain the tomatoes and chop.

Steam-fry the onion and garlic in a medium nonstick frying pan until they are soft and browned, adding stock as necessary to keep them from sticking.

Add the beans, vinegar or lemon juice, parsley and salt to the pan and mash the mixture with a potato masher. Stir in the chopped tomatoes, thyme, marjoram or basil and white pepper.

If you're serving the spread warm, stir it until it is quite hot, then transfer to a serving bowl and serve immediately.

MAKES 350 ml (12 fl oz)

Per 60 ml (2 fl oz): 73 calories/306 kJ, 4 g protein, 14 g carbohydrates, 2 g sugar, 0.5 g total fat, 3% calories from fat, 4 g fibre, 207 mg sodium

Red Wine Vinaigrette

This is a good basic dressing for many types of salads. Unlike plain juice or water, the oil substitute will help the dressing stick to the greens.

Fat-Free Oil Substitute

240 ml (8 fl oz) cold water
1 tablespoon low-sodium vegetarian stock powder
2 teaspoons cornflour

Dressing

300 ml (10 fl oz) Fat-Free Oil Substitute
60 ml (2 fl oz) red wine vinegar
1 tablespoon balsamic vinegar
1 clove garlic, crushed
1 teaspoon salt
1 tablespoon Dijon mustard (optional)
1 tablespoon brown sugar (optional)

For the oil substitute: Place the water in a small saucepan and whisk in the stock powder and cornflour. Cook over medium-high heat, stirring constantly, until thickened and clear.

For the dressing: Whisk, shake or blend the oil substitute, red wine and balsamic vinegars, garlic, salt, mustard, if desired, and sugar, if desired, until well mixed. Transfer to a jar and refrigerate.

MAKES 350 ml (12 fl oz)

Per 2 tablespoons: 6 calories/25 kJ, 0.5 g protein, 2 g carbohydrates, 0 g sugar, 0 g total fat, 0% calories from fat, 0.5 g fibre, 160 mg sodium

Variation

Balsamic Vinaigrette: Omit the red wine vinegar and use 5 tablespoons balsamic vinegar. Use the optional mustard and brown sugar.

Per 2 tablespoons: 11 calories/46 kJ, 0.5 g protein, 3 g carbohydrates, 1 g sugar, 0.5 g total fat, 3% calories from fat, 0.5 g fibre, 176 mg sodium

Fennel and Soya Parmesan Vinaigrette

A delicious and unusual salad dressing you can whip up in your blender.

240 ml (8 fl oz) Fat-Free Oil Substitute for Salad Dressings
    (page 203)
60 ml (2 fl oz) balsamic vinegar
2 tablespoons vegan parmesan cheese or nutritional yeast
1 teaspoon fennel seeds
¾ teaspoon salt
1 clove garlic
Freshly ground black pepper to taste

Combine Fat-Free Oil Substitute, vinegar, vegan parmesan or nutritional yeast, fennel seeds, salt, garlic and black pepper in a blender or with a hand blender. Refrigerate, and shake before using.

MAKES 300 ml (½ pt)

Per 2 generous tablespoons: 15 calories/63 kJ, 1 g protein, 3 g carbohydrates, 0 g sugar, 0 g total fat, 1% calories from fat, 0.5 g fibre, 160 mg sodium

Low-Fat Pesto

This delicious pesto keeps in the refrigerator for a couple of weeks or the freezer for up to six months. The lemon juice helps preserve the basil's bright green colour.

2 × 25 g packs fresh basil leaves
4 cloves garlic
200 g (7 oz) reduced-fat extra-firm silken tofu
5 tablespoons soya parmesan
1 tsp salt
½ tablespoon lemon juice (optional)

Place basil, garlic, tofu, soya parmesan, salt and lemon juice, if using, in the food processor and process until a paste forms. Place in a tightly covered container and refrigerate until ready to use.

The top may darken a little, but this is just oxidation and doesn't affect taste or nutrition – just stir the mixture.

When using on pasta, thin the pesto out with some of the hot pasta cooking water before mixing with the pasta.

If you like, freeze portions in ice cube trays or in small servings on a baking sheet, then put the frozen portions in a plastic bag in the freezer.

Note: If you don't have soya parmesan, you can either use 2 tablespoons light miso and omit the salt, or use 4 tablespoons nutritional yeast flakes and double the lemon juice.

MAKES 350 ml (12 fl oz)

Per 60 ml (2 fl oz): 53 calories/222 kJ, 5 g protein, 5 g carbohydrates, 0.5 g sugar, 0.5 g total fat, 5% calories from fat, 1 g fibre, 343 mg sodium

Creamy Poppy Seed Dressing

This quick and easy dressing is very low in fat. With just the right amount of sweetness, it's great on fruit salads and spinach salads.

230 g (8 oz) reduced-fat firm or extra-firm silken tofu,
    crumbled
180 ml (6 fl oz) apple juice
6 tablespoons reduced-fat soya milk
3 tablespoons cider vinegar
1 tablespoon poppy seeds
1½ tablespoons chopped onion
1½ tablespoons Dijon mustard
1 scant teaspoon salt

Place all the ingredients in a blender and process until smooth. Transfer to a jar and refrigerate. Shake before serving.

MAKES 480 ml (16 fl oz)

Per 60 ml (2 fl oz) serving: 45 calories/188 kJ, 3 g protein, 7 g carbohydrates, 1 g sugar, 1 g total fat, 18% calories from fat, 0.5 g fibre, 268 mg sodium

Creamy Black Pepper Dressing

This is sure to be a favourite, especially if you are a fan of spinach salads. The blender is the key to the creamy texture.

1½ tablespoons low-sodium vegetarian stock powder
340 g (12 oz) reduced-fat firm silken tofu
1 large clove garlic, finely chopped
3 tablespoons fresh lemon juice
1 tablespoon rice vinegar
1 tablespoon nutritional yeast flakes
1½ teaspoons whole black peppercorns
1 teaspoon miso
1 teaspoon sugar
¾ teaspoon salt
180 ml (6 fl oz) water

Place all the ingredients in a blender and process until very smooth. Transfer to a jar and refrigerate. Shake well before serving.

MAKES 480 ml (16 fl oz)

Per 2 tablespoons: 15 calories/63 kJ, 2 g protein, 2 g carbohydrates, 0.5 g sugar, 0.5 g total fat, 11% calories from fat, 0.5 g fibre, 123 mg sodium

Soups

Dutch Green Pea Soup

A very satisfying meal on a cold day! Serve this soup hot along with dark pumpernickel bread.

230 g (8 oz) green split peas
2 litres (3½ pt) low-sodium vegetarian stock
1 tablespoon vegetarian bacon bits
2 medium new potatoes, peeled and chopped
2 medium leeks, chopped, including any tender green parts
1 large celery stick, including leaves, chopped
½ teaspoon dried savory or thyme
285–340 g (10–12 oz) low-fat vegetarian hot dogs or sausages, sliced diagonally into chunks
Salt to taste
Freshly ground black pepper to taste

Bring the split peas, stock and bacon bits to the boil in a large saucepan, skimming off any foam. Reduce the heat, cover and simmer for about 3 hours. Add the potatoes, leeks, celery, savory, if desired, and hot dogs or sausages. Simmer for 30 minutes or until the potatoes are tender. Season with the salt and pepper.

MAKES 8 SERVINGS

Per serving: 184 calories/770 kJ, 15 g protein, 27 g carbohydrates, 3 g sugar, 3 g total fat, 11% calories from fat, 7 g fibre, 36 mg sodium

Barley and Winter Squash Soup

This is a lovely soup for a cold evening.

1 litre (1¾ pt) low-sodium vegetarian stock
455 g (1 lb) winter squash, i.e. acorn, peeled, seeded and cut into
   2 cm (¾ in) cubes
½ large onion, chopped
170 g (6 oz) low-fat chicken substitute pieces
150 g (5½ oz) pearl barley
230 g (8 oz) red potatoes, chopped
30 g (1 oz) chopped celery
1½ teaspoons vegetarian bacon bits
1 bay leaf
½ teaspoon dried thyme
½ teaspoon dried savory
350 ml (12 fl oz) reduced-fat soya milk
Salt to taste
Freshly ground black pepper to taste
Chopped fresh parsley (optional)

Place the stock, squash, onion, chicken substitute pieces, barley, potatoes, celery, bacon bits, bay leaf, thyme and savory in a soup pot and
bring to the boil. Reduce the heat to low, cover and simmer for 30
minutes. Remove the bay leaf, stir in the soya milk and season with the
salt and pepper. Sprinkle with chopped parsley, if desired.

MAKES 6 SERVINGS

Per serving: 204 calories/854 kJ, 11 g protein, 40 g carbohydrates, 4 g sugar, 1 g total fat,
4% calories from fat, 8 g fibre, 229 mg sodium

Creamy Mushroom Soup

A food processor turns this dairy-free soup into a rich, creamy treat
with a delightful mushroom flavour.

1 small onion, finely chopped
1.2 litres (2 pt) mushroom or vegetable stock

1 bay leaf
½ teaspoon dried thyme
100 g (3½ oz) rolled oats
340 g (12 oz) mushrooms, sliced
2 teaspoons low-sodium soy sauce
2 tablespoons dry sherry (optional)
Salt to taste
Freshly ground black pepper to taste
Vegan Parmesan cheese (optional)

Steam-fry the onion in a heavy nonstick frying pan over medium heat until soft but not browned, adding very small amounts of water as needed to prevent sticking and burning. (Or place in a microwaveable dish, cover and microwave on high for 3 minutes.)

Place the stock, bay leaf, thyme and oats in a medium saucepan. Add the onion and bring to the boil, then reduce the heat to low, cover and simmer for 20 minutes or until the oats are soft.

Meanwhile, steam-fry the mushrooms in a large, heavy nonstick frying pan over high heat, adding a sprinkle of salt and very small amounts of water as needed to prevent sticking and burning. Cook until the mushrooms release and reabsorb their liquid. Remove from the heat and set aside.

When the oats are soft, remove the bay leaf and purée the soup until creamy with a hand-held blender or in batches in a blender or food processor. (Remove the middle part of the blender or food processor's lid so hot air can escape. Cover the hole loosely with a folded clean cloth while blending.)

Return the soup to the pan and add the mushrooms, soy sauce, sherry (if desired), salt, pepper and vegan Parmesan (if desired). Serve hot.

MAKES 4 SERVINGS

Per serving: 80 calories/335 kJ, 5 g protein, 14 g carbohydrates, 3 g sugar, 1 g total fat, 12% calories from fat, 3 g fibre, 93 mg sodium

Black-Eyed Bean and Sweet Potato Soup

Delicious, hearty ingredients – black-eyed beans, vegetarian bacon and sausage, sweet potatoes and greens – make this soup very satisfying.

1 large onion, chopped
3 cloves garlic, crushed
1.5 litres (2½ pt) low-sodium vegetarian stock
4 tablespoons tomato purée
2 × 420 g tins black-eyed beans, rinsed and drained
2 tablespoons vegetarian bacon bits
2 teaspoons dried oregano
1 bay leaf
½ teaspoon salt
½ teaspoon dried crushed chillies
115 g (4 oz) kale or other dark greens, cleaned, trimmed and
   thinly sliced
455 g (1 lb) sweet potatoes, peeled and chopped
2 vegetarian sausages, cut into 5 mm (¼ in) slices

Steam-fry the onion and garlic in a large, heavy nonstick frying pan over medium heat until soft, adding very small amounts of water as needed to prevent sticking and burning. (Or place in a microwaveable dish, cover and microwave on high for 5 minutes.)

Place the stock, tomato purée, black-eyed beans, bacon bits, oregano, bay leaf, salt, crushed chillies, greens, sweet potatoes and sausage in a large saucepan. Add the onion and garlic and simmer for 30 minutes or until the sweet potatoes are tender. Remove the bay leaf and serve immediately.

MAKES 6 SERVINGS

Per serving: 257 calories/1076 kJ, 16 g protein, 44 g carbohydrates, 8 g sugar, 3 g total fat, 10% calories from fat, 10 g fibre, 263 mg sodium

Red Lentil and Sweet Potato Soup

This hearty soup makes a great light lunch or a starter for a several-course meal. Blending gives it a delightfully smooth texture.

2 small onions, chopped
½ teaspoon ground cumin
½ teaspoon ground ginger
1 litre (1¾ pt) low-sodium vegetarian stock
2 medium sweet potatoes, peeled and cubed
125 g (4½ oz) red or pink lentils, rinsed
1 teaspoon lemon juice
¼ teaspoon salt
White pepper to taste
Paprika

Steam-fry the onions in a large, heavy nonstick frying pan over medium heat until soft, adding very small amounts of water as needed to prevent sticking and burning. (Or place in a microwave-able dish, cover and microwave on high for 5 minutes.) Stir in the cumin and ginger and blend well.

Place the stock, sweet potatoes and lentils in a medium soup pot. Add the onions and simmer, uncovered, for about 30 minutes or until the lentils are tender. Add the lemon juice, salt and white pepper. Process using a hand-held blender in the pan or in batches in a blender or food processor, until creamy. (Remove the middle part of the blender or food processor lid so hot air can escape. Cover the hole loosely with a folded clean cloth while blending.) Serve hot and with paprika sprinkled on top of each bowl.

MAKES 4 SERVINGS

Per serving: 185 calories/774 kJ, 10 g protein, 36 g carbohydrates, 4 g sugar, 1 g total fat, 3% calories from fat, 6 g fibre, 158 mg sodium

Sandwiches and Salads

Black Bean Soft Tacos

In Mexico, tacos are usually made with fresh, hot tortillas (not deep-fried ones). This machine-blended filling brings you all the traditional taste and heartiness of the real thing. Recently, black beans have become much more widely available so you should be able to find them in your local supermarket.

Tofu Soured Cream

340 g (12 oz) reduced-fat extra-firm silken tofu, crumbled
3 tablespoons lemon juice
½ teaspoon sugar
¼ teaspoon salt

Tacos

8 × 15 cm (6 in) corn tortillas
375 g (13 oz) Vegetarian 'Refried' Beans made with black beans
  (page 199)
1 recipe Low-Fat Guacamole (page 198)
170 g (6 oz) no-sugar-added tomato salsa
275 g (9¼ oz) finely shredded green cabbage or lettuce
240 ml (8 fl oz) Tofu Soured Cream

For the tofu soured cream: Place the tofu, lemon juice, sugar and salt in a food processor or blender and process until very smooth. Refrigerate in a covered container for up to 1 week.

For the tacos: Heat the tortillas (see Note). Spread about 3 tablespoons of beans down the middle of each tortilla. Top with guacamole, salsa, cabbage or lettuce and tofu soured cream.

Note: If the tortillas are frozen, heat them between two microwaveable plates on high for about 1 minute, then turn over the plates and heat for 1 minute longer. You can soften thawed or fresh tortillas in a hot, dry pan; grill them quickly just until soft; or wrap them in a clean kitchen towel moistened with hot water, then wrap them in foil and bake them in a 180°C/350°F/gas 4 oven for about 12 minutes.

MAKES 8 SERVINGS

Per serving: 174 calories/728 kJ, 10 g protein, 33 g carbohydrates, 3 g sugar, 1 g total fat, 7% calories from fat, 7 g fibre, 557 mg sodium

Asparagus and Veggie Ham Panini

2 slices rye or sprouted-grain bread
2 tablespoons Tofu Mayonnaise (page 222)
6 thin asparagus spears, steamed or roasted
6 fresh basil leaves
2 slices low-fat vegetarian bacon or ham

Spread each bread slice on 1 side with 1 tablespoon Tofu Mayonnaise and assemble the sandwich with the rest of the ingredients the way you like it, being careful not to overfill.

The easiest way to make panini is with an electric sandwich toaster or mini grill. Set the timer for 5 minutes, then check the bread. If it is not as golden and crisp as you like, cook for a few minutes longer. Cut the sandwich into triangles and serve hot.

If you do not have a sandwich toaster or mini grill, cook the sandwich in a heavy nonstick frying pan or on a griddle over medium heat, pressing down on the sandwich with a fish slice as you brown each side.

Per serving (using rye bread): 308 calories/1289 kJ, 31 g protein, 32 g carbohydrates, 0.2 g sugar, 4 g total fat, 11% calories from fat, 6 g fibre, 825 mg sodium

Italian Stuffed Griddle Dumplings

This traditional 'griddle dumpling' from Romagna is actually a stuffed Italian flatbread, similar to a calzone but stuffed with greens. This easy version uses wholemeal pittas.

6 wholemeal pittas
230 g (8 oz) Swiss chard, spinach or savoy cabbage, or a mixture
230 g (8 oz) bitter greens, such as rocket, radicchio or curly
    endive
1½ teaspoons chopped garlic
60 ml (2 fl oz) low-sodium vegetable stock
¼ teaspoon salt plus extra to taste
Freshly ground black pepper to taste

Cut the pittas in half and open to form a pocket. Wash, trim and thinly slice the greens.

Place the garlic, stock, greens and salt in a large, deep nonstick frying pan. Bring to the boil, then cover, reduce the heat to medium and cook until tender. If any liquid remains, uncover and cook over high heat, stirring constantly, until it evaporates. Season with the salt and pepper and set aside to cool.

Drain the greens and stuff inside the pitta halves. Heat the filled pittas on a hot, dry griddle or cast-iron pan over high heat, turning frequently, until hot and flecked with brown spots. Serve hot.

MAKES 6 SERVINGS

Per serving: 188 calories/787 kJ, 8 g protein, 38 g carbohydrates, 2 g sugar, 2 g total fat, 8% calories from fat, 6 g fibre, 510 mg sodium

Mediterranean Veggie Panini

Italian sandwich making has become an art form in the northern city of Milan and has spread all over Europe and North America. Sandwich bars in Italy range from humble places to the height of sophistication, and some offer as many as 30 varieties.

2 slices rye or sprouted-grain bread
2 tablespoons fat-free Italian vinaigrette dressing
2 jarred roasted red peppers, rinsed and patted dry
60 g (2 oz) tender kale leaves or other greens
2 small firm, ripe tomatoes, sliced
75 g (2½ oz) sliced marinated artichoke hearts, rinsed, drained
    and patted dry

Moisten each bread slice on 1 side with 1 tablespoon dressing and assemble the sandwich with the rest of the ingredients the way you like it, being careful not to overfill.

The easiest way to make panini is with an electric sandwich toaster or mini grill. Set the timer for 5 minutes, then check the bread. If it is not as golden and crisp as you like, cook for a few minutes longer. Cut the sandwich into triangles and serve hot.

If you do not have a sandwich toaster or grill, cook the sandwich in a heavy nonstick frying pan or on a griddle over medium heat, pressing down on the sandwich with a fish slice as you brown each side.

MAKES 1 SERVING

Per serving (using rye bread): 311 calories/1302 kJ, 13 g protein, 49 g carbohydrates, 4.9 g sugar, 3 g fat, 8% calories from fat, 13.3 g fibre, 849 mg sodium

Thai-Style Coleslaw

This easy coleslaw makes a great winter accompaniment to a spicy meal or spices up any other meal.

250 g (9 oz) finely shredded green or savoy cabbage
1 medium carrot, grated
1 small sweet onion, thinly sliced
2 tablespoons finely chopped fresh mint or 2 teaspoons dried
   mint
2 tablespoons finely chopped fresh coriander, basil or parsley
2 tablespoons low-sodium soy sauce
2 tablespoons lime juice
2 tablespoons water
1 tablespoon sugar
1 tablespoon grated lime peel
1½ teaspoons toasted sesame seeds

Combine the cabbage, carrot, onion, mint and coriander, basil or parsley in a serving bowl.

Combine the soy sauce, lime juice, water, sugar and lime peel in a small bowl. Pour over the salad, mix well and refrigerate until ready to serve. Sprinkle with the sesame seeds before serving.

MAKES 4 SERVINGS

Per serving: 61 calories/255 kJ, 2 g protein, 13 g carbohydrates, 8 g sugar, 1 g total fat, 10% calories from fat, 3 g fibre, 334 mg sodium

Orange Quinoa and Bulgur Tabbouleh

This is a delicious and unusual version of the well-known Middle Eastern salad.

90 g (3 oz) medium-grain bulgur wheat
350 ml (12 fl oz) water
90 g (3 oz) quinoa
180 ml (6 fl oz) Fat-Free Oil Substitute (page 203)

60 ml (2 fl oz) lemon juice
1 teaspoon salt
1 teaspoon ground coriander
2 pinches ground cinnamon
Freshly ground black pepper to taste
115 g (4 oz) chopped fresh parsley
170 g (6 oz) cooked or tinned black-eyed beans, rinsed and
  drained
1 chopped, seeded green pepper
8 tablespoons chopped fresh mint or lemon balm
50 g (1¾ oz) chopped spring onion
Grated peel of 2 oranges
4 jarred roasted red peppers, rinsed and chopped
Orange wedges (optional)
Mint, parsley or lemon balm sprigs (optional)

Soak the bulgur in 120 ml (4 fl oz) boiling water in a large bowl, covered, for 30 minutes. Meanwhile, bring the quinoa and 240 ml (8 fl oz) water to the boil in a small saucepan. Reduce the heat to low, cover, and cook for 15 minutes. Remove from the heat and let stand until the bulgur is ready.

Whisk or blend together the oil substitute, lemon juice, salt, coriander, cinnamon and black pepper in a small bowl. Set aside.

Combine the quinoa with the bulgur. Add the parsley, black-eyed beans, green pepper, mint or lemon balm, spring onion, orange peel, red peppers and oil dressing and mix well. Garnish with orange wedges and sprigs of mint, parsley or lemon balm, if desired. Refrigerate, but let stand at room temperature for 30 minutes before serving.

MAKES 8 SERVINGS

Per serving: 136 calories/569 kJ, 5 g protein, 29 g carbohydrates, 2 g sugar, 1 g total fat, 7% calories from fat, 7 g fibre, 303 mg sodium

Cherry Tomato and Brown Rice Salad with Artichoke Hearts

This delicious salad is a complete meal and a great picnic or barbecue dish. Because neither tomatoes nor rice benefit from refrigeration, it should served at room temperature.

570 g (1¼ lb) cooked brown basmati rice, warm
170 g (6 oz) marinated artichoke hearts, rinsed in hot water,
  drained and sliced
100 g (3½ oz) chopped spring onions
685 g (1½ lb) red, yellow or mixed cherry tomatoes, halved
20 g (¾ oz) chopped fresh basil
120 ml (4 fl oz) fat-free Italian dressing
3 tablespoons lemon juice
2 cloves garlic, crushed
¼ teaspoon salt
Freshly ground black pepper to taste
1 head crisp lettuce

Place the rice in a large salad bowl and add the artichokes, spring onions, tomatoes and basil. Mix gently.

Combine the Italian dressing, lemon juice, garlic, salt and pepper in a small bowl or jar. Whisk or shake until well blended. Pour over the salad and mix gently. Serve on beds of lettuce on individual plates.

MAKES 6 SERVINGS

Per serving: 153 calories/640 kJ, 4 g protein, 32 g carbohydrates, 3 g sugar, 1 g total fat, 6% calories from fat, 4 g fibre, 376 mg sodium

Mixed Bean Salad

This quick and delicious salad keeps for up to a week in the refrigerator for quick lunches or a hearty addition to a green salad. It is not only free of oil, but contains much less sugar than typical bean salads found in supermarkets.

420 g tin chickpeas, rinsed and drained
420 g tin red kidney beans, rinsed and drained
420 g tin black-eyed beans, rinsed and drained
170 g (6 oz) cooked fresh or frozen green beans
2 medium sticks celery, diced
1 large pepper, any colour, chopped
3 spring onions, chopped
5 tablespoons finely chopped parsley
240 ml (8 fl oz) Fat-Free Oil Substitute (page 203)
150 ml (5 fl oz) red wine vinegar
3 tablespoons sugar or maple syrup
3 cloves garlic, crushed
1 teaspoon salt
1 teaspoon dry mustard powder
Freshly ground black pepper to taste

Mix the chickpeas, kidney beans, black-eyed beans, green beans, celery, chopped pepper, spring onions and parsley in a serving bowl. Blend the oil substitute, vinegar, sugar or maple syrup, garlic, salt, mustard powder and black pepper. Pour over the salad. Mix well. Cover and store in the refrigerator.

MAKES 8 SERVINGS

Per serving: 172 calories/720 kJ, 9 g protein, 33 g carbohydrates, 8 g sugar, 1 g total fat, 5% calories from fat, 9 g fibre, 332 mg sodium

Red Cabbage Slaw with Cranberries and Apples

This is a very easy, attractive and delicious make-ahead salad for winter meals. A blender makes the vinaigrette in a jiffy.

Cranberry-Orange Vinaigrette
180 ml (6 fl oz) Fat-Free Oil Substitute (page 203)
120 ml (4 fl oz) orange juice
30 g (1 oz) chopped fresh or frozen cranberries
2 tablespoons red wine vinegar
1½ tablespoons chopped chives or spring onion
1 tablespoon balsamic vinegar
1 tablespoon lemon juice
1 tablespoon sugar
1 large clove garlic, crushed
1 teaspoon salt
Freshly ground black pepper to taste

Salad
685 g (1½ lb) red cabbage, thinly sliced
75 g (2½ oz) fresh or frozen cranberries
2 crisp sweet apples, sliced

For the vinaigrette: Blend the oil substitute, orange juice, cranberries, wine vinegar, chives or spring onion, balsamic vinegar, lemon juice, sugar, garlic, salt and pepper in a blender. If making ahead, transfer to a covered container and refrigerate.

For the salad: Combine the cabbage, cranberries and vinaigrette in a medium salad bowl and toss gently. Cover and refrigerate for at least 2 hours to allow the flavours to blend. When ready to serve, slice the apples (with peel), add to the salad and toss well.

MAKES 8 SERVINGS

Per serving: 70 calories/293 kJ, 1 g protein, 18 g carbohydrates, 11 g sugar, 0.5 g total fat, 2% calories from fat, 3 g fibre, 251 mg sodium

Sautéed Portabella Mushroom Salad

This is a very simple and delicious salad for two.

150 g (5½ oz) mixed baby salad greens
60 ml (2 fl oz) Fat-Free Oil Substitute (page 203)
2 tablespoons balsamic vinegar
1 teaspoon Dijon mustard
¼ teaspoon salt
¼ teaspoon coarsely ground black pepper
2 large portabella mushrooms
Wine or vegetable stock
4 spring onions, sliced

Divide the greens between two serving plates. In a small bowl, whisk together the oil substitute, vinegar, mustard, salt and pepper. Set aside.

Remove the stems from the mushrooms and scrape away the dark gills with the edge of a spoon.

Heat a large, heavy nonstick frying pan over high heat and add the mushrooms. Cover and cook until slightly browned on the bottoms and beginning to release a bit of liquid. Add a very small amount of wine or stock as needed to prevent sticking. Turn the mushrooms and brown the other side.

Quickly slice the mushrooms and place them evenly over the greens. Drizzle with the dressing, sprinkle with the spring onions and serve immediately.

MAKES 2 SERVINGS

Per serving: 95 calories/398 kJ, 7 g protein, 19 g carbohydrates, 4 g sugar, 1 g total fat, 6% calories from fat, 7 g fibre, 308 mg sodium

BLT Salad

A salad version of the well-loved sandwich that uses a handy mayonnaise substitute. Cooks, plug in your blenders!

Tofu Mayonnaise
340 g (12 oz) reduced-fat extra-firm silken tofu
2 tablespoons cider vinegar or lemon juice
1⅛ teaspoons salt
½ teaspoon dry mustard
⅛ teaspoon white pepper

Salad
1 large romaine lettuce, torn into pieces
340 g (12 oz) cubed sprouted-wheat bread, lightly toasted
4 slices low-fat vegetarian bacon
360 g (12½ oz) ripe firm tomatoes, chopped
2 spring onions, sliced
120 ml (4 fl oz) cider vinegar
80 ml (3 fl oz) Fat-Free Oil Substitute (page 203)
60 ml (2 fl oz) Tofu Mayonnaise
5 teaspoons sugar
Freshly ground black pepper to taste

For the mayonnaise: Combine the tofu, vinegar or lemon juice, salt, mustard and pepper in a food processor or blender (or place the ingredients in a medium bowl and use a hand-held blender) and process until very smooth. It will keep in a covered container in the refrigerator for about 2 weeks.

For the salad: Combine the lettuce, bread cubes, bacon, tomatoes and spring onions in a large bowl.

Whisk together the vinegar, oil substitute, tofu mayonnaise, sugar and pepper in a medium bowl until well blended. Toss with the salad. Divide the salad evenly among 4 salad bowls or plates and serve immediately.

MAKES 4 SERVINGS

Per serving: 259 calories/1084 kJ, 13 g protein, 42 g carbohydrates, 11 g sugar, 2 g total fat, 8% calories from fat, 10 g fibre, 639 mg sodium

Main Courses

Savoury Soya Roast

You'll find this dish firmer and more appetizing if you let it cool thoroughly, then slice and reheat it. I make it early in the day or the day before I plan to eat it. It is especially good with Rich Brown Gravy (page 224), or just ketchup.

1 litre (1¾ pt) low-sodium vegetable stock
60 ml (2 fl oz) low-sodium ketchup
2 tablespoons low-sodium soy sauce
75 g (2½ oz) dry textured soya protein granules (soya mince)
75 g (2½ oz) oat bran
2 tablespoons ground flaxseed
1 tablespoon nutritional yeast flakes
1 teaspoon garlic granules
1 teaspoon onion powder
1 teaspoon dried thyme (or other herb of choice)
Freshly ground black pepper to taste
120 ml (4 fl oz) low-sodium tomato sauce, ketchup or barbecue
    sauce

Preheat the oven to 190°C/375°F/gas 5.

Pour the stock into a medium bowl, add the ketchup, soy sauce and textured soya protein and let the mixture stand 5 to 10 minutes, or until all of the liquid is absorbed.

Add the oat bran, flaxseed, nutritional yeast flakes, garlic granules, onion powder, thyme and black pepper. Mix well and pack into a

22 × 12 cm (9 × 5 in) loaf tin, lined on the bottom with baking parchment.

Spread the tomato sauce, ketchup or barbecue sauce over the top evenly. Bake for 45 minutes. Let the soya roast cool thoroughly in the refrigerator before slicing. Reheat, if necessary, in the micro-wave, or wrapped in foil in a 180°C/350°F/gas 4 oven for 20 to 25 minutes.

MAKES 6 SERVINGS

Per serving: 190 calories/795 kJ, 18 g protein, 31 g carbohydrates, 10 g sugar, 3 g total fat, 10% calories from fat, 4 g fibre, 219 mg sodium

Rich Brown Gravy

This fat-free and delicious brown gravy will become a favourite staple. If you can't find oat flour in your local health food store grind old-fashioned or quick-cooking oats in a dry blender or electric coffee/spice mill.

3 tablespoons nutritional yeast flakes
2 tablespoons oat flour
4 tablespoons chickpea flour (besan)
600 ml (1 pt) water
2 tablespoons low-sodium soy sauce
½ teaspoon salt
a few shakes of gravy browner (optional)

In a heavy saucepan over high heat, whisk the nutritional yeast flakes and flours together until it smells toasty. Off the heat, whisk in the water, soy sauce, salt and gravy browner, if using. (You can use a hand blender to do this, if you wish.) Stir constantly over high heat until it thickens and comes to the boil. Reduce the heat and simmer for 2 to 5 minutes. This can be made ahead and reheated.

MAKES 600 ml (1 pt)

Per 60 ml (2 fl oz): 27 calories/113 kJ, 3 g protein, 4 g carbohydrates, 0.5 g sugar, 0.5 g total fat, 13% calories from fat, 1 g fibre, 218 mg sodium

White Bean and Sweet Potato Stew

All you need is wholemeal bread to go with this Italian-inspired stew.

1 large onion, chopped
4 cloves garlic, chopped
2 × 420 g tins cannellini or other white beans, rinsed and
  drained
2 × 400 g tins low-sodium diced tomatoes
455 g (1 lb) sweet potatoes, peeled and cut into 2 cm (¾ in)
  cubes
230 g (8 oz) cremini mushrooms, sliced
240 ml (8 fl oz) low-sodium vegetarian stock
120–180 ml (4–6 fl oz) dry red wine
1 tablespoon vegetarian bacon bits
1 teaspoon salt
1 teaspoon each dried rosemary, thyme and basil
1 bay leaf
¼ teaspoon dried crushed chillies
340 g (12 oz) kale, thinly sliced
Salt and freshly ground black pepper to taste

Steam-fry the onion and garlic in a large, heavy nonstick saucepan over medium heat until soft, adding very small amounts of water, wine or stock as needed to prevent sticking and burning. (Or place in a microwaveable dish, cover and microwave on high power for 5 minutes.)

Add the beans, tomatoes (with juice), sweet potatoes, mushrooms, stock, wine, bacon bits, salt, rosemary, thyme, basil, bay leaf and crushed chillies to the pan. Simmer for 35 to 40 minutes until the sauce is thick and the sweet potato cooked. Meanwhile, steam the kale and stir into the stew 5 minutes before the end of cooking. To serve, remove the bay leaf and season with the salt and pepper.

MAKES 6 SERVINGS

Per serving: 257 calories/1075 kJ, 14 g protein, 50 g carbohydrates, 9 g sugar, 2 g total fat, 4% calories from fat, 12 g fibre, 418 mg sodium

Lebanese-Style Lentils and Pasta

This delicious Lebanese dish makes a full meal.

1.2 litres (2 pt) low-sodium vegetable stock
200 g (7 oz) uncooked brown lentils, rinsed
2 medium onions, chopped
2 cloves garlic, chopped
1 teaspoon ground cumin
275 g (9¼ oz) chopped chard, kale or other greens or 285 g
   (10 oz) frozen chopped spinach, thawed and squeezed dry
115 g (4 oz) spaghetti (preferably wholewheat), broken into
   10 cm (4 in) long pieces
4 tablespoons chopped fresh parsley or coriander (optional)
Pinch of cayenne pepper
2 tablespoons lemon juice
Salt to taste
Freshly ground black pepper to taste

Bring the stock and lentils to the boil in a medium saucepan. Reduce the heat to low, cover and cook for about 25 minutes or until the lentils are tender but still hold their shape.

Steam-fry the onions, garlic and cumin in a large, heavy nonstick saucepan or deep frying pan until soft, adding very small amounts of water as needed to prevent sticking and burning. (Or place in a microwaveable dish, cover and microwave on high for 7 minutes.)

Pour the lentils and stock into the pan with the onions. Add the greens, pasta, parsley or coriander, if desired, and cayenne. Bring to the boil, then reduce the heat to medium. Cook, uncovered, for about 10 minutes or until the pasta is tender and most of the stock has been absorbed, leaving a sauce. Add the lemon juice and mix well. Season with the salt and black pepper. Serve hot.

MAKES 4 SERVINGS

Per serving: 318 calories/1331 kJ, 20 g protein, 61 g carbohydrates, 7 g sugar, 1 g total fat, 3% calories from fat, 17 g fibre, 204 mg sodium

Lemon and Artichoke Tagine

Serve this delicious stew with Bulgur Wheat and Quinoa Pilaf (page 236) and a crisp green salad.

2 tablespoons wholemeal flour
340 g (12 oz) low-fat chicken substitute pieces
1 large onion, sliced
6 cloves garlic, chopped
145 g (5 oz) sliced mushrooms
1 large green or red pepper, cored, seeded and cut into chunks
480 ml (16 fl oz) low-sodium vegetarian stock
1 tablespoon ground coriander
1 tablespoon dried parsley
½ teaspoon black pepper
¼ teaspoon ground turmeric
¼ teaspoon ground ginger
¼ teaspoon paprika
¼ teaspoon dried crushed chillies
1 lemon, with peel, sliced and seeded
200 g (7 oz) jar marinated artichoke heart quarters, rinsed under
    hot water and drained
Salt to taste

Place the flour in a shallow dish and roll the chicken substitute pieces to coat. Place the pieces in a large, heavy, deep nonstick frying pan over medium-high heat and cook until browned. Remove from the pan and set aside.

Add the onion and garlic to the pan and steam-fry until soft, adding very small amounts of water as needed to prevent sticking and burning. (Or place in a microwaveable dish, cover and microwave on high for 7 minutes.)

Add the chicken substitute pieces, mushrooms, pepper, stock, coriander, parsley, black pepper, turmeric, ginger, paprika and crushed chillies. Place the lemon slices on top of the stew, cover, reduce the heat and simmer for 30 minutes.

Remove and discard the lemon slices. Stir in the artichokes and cook just until heated. Season with the salt and serve immediately.

MAKES 4 SERVINGS

Per serving: 165 calories/691 kJ, 20 g protein, 25 g carbohydrates, 3 g sugar, 1 g total fat, 3% calories from fat, 10 g fibre, 584 mg sodium

Pasta with Lentil and Tomato Sauce

455 g (1 lb) pasta of choice
Family size (750 g) jar fat-free tomato sauce for pasta
420 g tin lentils, rinsed and drained
120 ml (4 fl oz) dry red wine or low-sodium vegetarian stock
Salt to taste
Freshly ground black pepper

Cook the pasta according to package directions, then drain.

Meanwhile, combine the pasta sauce, lentils and wine or stock in a medium saucepan. Heat gently and season with the salt and pepper. Serve over the pasta.

MAKES 5 SERVINGS

Per serving: 470 calories/1967 kJ, 19 g protein, 91 g carbohydrates, 9 g sugar, 2 g total fat, 3% calories from fat, 8 g fibre, 173 mg sodium

Vegetarian Mixed-Bean Chilli

This chilli is an absolutely delicious savoury treat. Serve it with brown basmati rice, sprouted-grain bread, corn tortillas or soft fresh polenta, and a salad. Leftovers freeze well.

6 cloves garlic, crushed
1 tablespoon chilli powder
1 tablespoon dried oregano
1½ teaspoons ground cumin
½ teaspoon dried crushed chillies
2 × 400 g tins chopped tomatoes
420 g tin borlotti beans, rinsed and drained
420 g tin black beans, rinsed and drained
420 g tin red kidney beans, rinsed and drained
700 ml (1¼ pt) hot water
60 g (2 oz) dry textured vegetable protein
200 g (7 oz) frozen sweetcorn
1 large green pepper, cored, seeded and chopped
60 ml (2 fl oz) low-sodium soy sauce
1 tablespoon hot pepper sauce
1 tablespoon onion powder
1 tablespoon unsweetened cocoa powder
1 teaspoon sugar
2 tablespoons cornmeal or masa harina
Salt to taste

Steam-fry the garlic in a large, heavy nonstick frying pan for 2 minutes. Add the chilli powder, oregano, cumin and crushed chillies and stir-fry for 1 minute. Add the tomatoes (with juice), beans, hot water, vegetable protein, sweetcorn, pepper, soy sauce, hot pepper sauce, onion powder, cocoa and sugar. Bring to the boil, then reduce the heat, cover and simmer for 15 to 30 minutes. During the last 5 minutes of cooking, sprinkle the cornmeal or masa harina over the top and stir in thoroughly. Season with the salt.

MAKES 6 SERVINGS

Per serving: 329 calories/1377 kJ, 26 g protein, 57 g carbohydrates, 7 g sugar, 2 g total fat, 4% calories from fat, 16 g fibre, 457 mg sodium

Indonesian-Style Stir-Fried Pasta

This dish has just the right exotic touch. If your local health food store doesn't stock soya spaghetti try Internet suppliers.

455 g (1 lb) soya spaghetti
1 medium onion, chopped
6 cloves garlic, crushed
½–1 teaspoon dried crushed chillies
145 g (5 oz) shredded savoy cabbage
2 celery sticks, sliced thinly on the diagonal
60 ml (2 fl oz) water
170 g (6 oz) low-fat beef or chicken substitute pieces
120 ml (4 fl oz) low-sodium vegetarian stock
60 ml (2 fl oz) low-sodium soy sauce
¾ tablespoon maple syrup
¾ tablespoon dark molasses
2 teaspoons cornflour
1 tablespoon cold water
4 spring onions, sliced thinly on the diagonal

Cook the pasta in a large pot of boiling water until tender. Drain in a colander.

In a large, heavy nonstick wok or a frying pan lightly coated with oil or cooking spray, steam-fry the onion, garlic and crushed chillies for 1 minute, adding very small amounts of water as needed to prevent sticking and burning.

Add the cabbage, celery and 60 ml (2 fl oz) water. Cover and cook over high heat for about 3 minutes. Add the beef substitute pieces and stir-fry for about 1 minute.

Combine the stock, soy sauce, maple syrup, molasses, cornflour and cold water in a small bowl. Stir into the pan and cook, stirring, over high heat until it thickens and boils.

Add the drained pasta and toss well with the sauce. Top with the spring onions and serve.

MAKES 6 SERVINGS

Per serving: 338 calories/1415 kJ, 10 g protein, 74 g carbohydrates, 19 g sugar, 1 g total fat, 2% calories from fat, 5 g fibre, 505 mg sodium

Quick Spinach Lasagne

Although it takes a little more than an hour to make this dish, most of that is cooking time; prep takes just a few minutes.

285 g (10 oz) frozen spinach, thawed
455 g (1 lb) reduced-fat firm tofu
1 tablespoon chopped or crushed garlic
1 teaspoon salt
Family size jar (750 g) fat-free tomato sauce for pasta
455 g (1 lb) lasagne sheets (preferably wholewheat)
10 button mushrooms, sliced
4 tablespoons vegan Parmesan or nutritional yeast flakes

Preheat the oven to 160°C/325°F/gas 3.

Combine the spinach, tofu, garlic and salt in a medium bowl.

Coat the bottom of a 23 × 32 cm (9 × 13 in) baking dish with tomato sauce, then add a layer of pasta, overlapping them slightly. Spread half of the spinach mixture over the pasta. Follow with another layer of pasta, then tomato sauce, and a layer of mushrooms. Repeat until the layers reach the top of the dish. The final layer should be sauce topped with vegan Parmesan or yeast flakes.

Cover tightly with foil and bake for 1 hour. Stick a knife through the centre of the lasagne to be sure the pasta is completely cooked. Let stand for 15 minutes, uncovered, before serving.

MAKES 8 SERVINGS

Per serving: 332 calories/1390 kJ, 18 g protein, 5 g carbohydrates, 7 g sugar, 5 g total fat, 9% calories from fat, 9 g fibre, 284 mg sodium

Adapted from a recipe by Jennifer Reilly

Aubergine Parmesan

This interpretation of an old favourite appeals to modern tastes, with 'béchamel' sauce and vegan Parmesan providing a creamy contrast.

Creamy Béchamel Sauce
½ medium onion, cut into chunks
240 ml (8 fl oz) water
150 g (5½ oz) cooked or tinned white beans, rinsed and drained
170 g (6 oz) reduced-fat firm silken tofu
1 tablespoon nutritional yeast flakes
1 teaspoon salt
¼ teaspoon dried garlic granules

Aubergine
1.4 kg (3 lb) aubergine, cut into 5-mm (¼-in) thick slices
75 g (2½ oz) fine dry breadcrumbs
700 ml (1¼ pt) fat-free tomato sauce for pasta
480 ml (16 fl oz) Creamy Béchamel Sauce
8 tablespoons vegan Parmesan

For the sauce: Simmer the onion with 240 ml (8 fl oz) water in a medium saucepan, covered, for about 10 minutes. Place in a blender or food processor with the remaining ingredients and blend until very smooth. The sauce can be refrigerated in a covered container for up to 1 week.

For the aubergine: Arrange the aubergine slices in a single layer on a nonstick baking sheet. Grill about 7 cm (3 in) from the heat on both sides until lightly browned and soft inside.

Preheat the oven to 160°C/325°F/gas 3. Lay half of the aubergine in the bottom of a 23 cm (10 in) round nonstick baking tin (or a baking tin lined with parchment) and top with half of the breadcrumbs. Spread with half of the pasta sauce, béchamel sauce and vegan Parmesan. Repeat with the remaining ingredients. Bake for 20 minutes, or until bubbly and browned on top.

MAKES 6 SERVINGS

Per serving: 262 calories/1097 kJ, 11 g protein, 34 g carbohydrates, 7 g sugar, 1 g total fat, 6% calories from fat, 10 g fibre, 697 mg sodium

Pasta with Chickpeas

2 litres (3½ pt) low-sodium vegetarian stock
2 × 420 g tins no-salt-added chickpeas, drained
3 carrots, chopped
230 g (8 oz) dried pasta shells (conchiglie)
3 cloves garlic, crushed (can be from a jar)
170 g (6 oz) chopped raw greens
Hot pepper sauce (optional)

Bring the stock to the boil in a large pot. Add the chickpeas, carrots, pasta, garlic and greens to the pot and turn down to a simmer. When the carrots and pasta are tender, the soup is ready. Ladle the soup into bowls and pass pepper sauce for those who like it hot.

MAKES 6 SERVINGS

Per serving: 306 calories/1281 kJ, 14 g protein, 58 g carbohydrates, 5 g sugar, 3 g total fat, 8% calories from fat, 9 g fibre, 44 mg sodium

Sides

Orange Couscous Pilaf

Couscous looks like a grain but is actually a type of semolina pasta that cooks quickly and makes a delicious side dish.

480 ml (16 fl oz) low-sodium vegetarian stock
145 g (5 oz) couscous
115 g (4 oz) carrots, grated
2 large oranges, peeled and cut into small chunks
4 teaspoons grated orange peel
2 tablespoons raisins
¼ teaspoon salt
¼ teaspoon ground cinnamon

Bring the stock and couscous to the boil in a large saucepan over high heat. Add the carrots, oranges, orange peel, raisins, salt and cinnamon. Return to the boil, then turn off the heat, cover and let stand for 10 minutes or until all liquid is absorbed. Fluff with a fork.

MAKES 4 SERVINGS

Per serving: 238 calories/996 kJ, 7 g protein, 52 g carbohydrates, 4 g sugar, 1 g total fat, 2% calories from fat, 7 g fibre, 143 mg sodium

Brussels Sprouts with Lemon and Vegetarian Bacon

This is a delicious and quick brussels sprout dish. You can partially cook the sprouts ahead of time, stop the cooking with ice water and then assemble and stir-fry the dish in minutes just before serving.

1.4 kg (3 lb) brussels sprouts, trimmed and halved vertically
8 slices vegetarian bacon, chopped
4 spring onions, chopped
60 ml (2 fl oz) low-sodium vegetarian stock
Salt to taste
Freshly ground black pepper to taste
2 tablespoons lemon juice

Add the brussels sprouts to a saucepan of boiling water and cook for 3 minutes. Drain immediately and plunge into ice-cold water to stop the cooking process. When they are cold, drain well.

Heat a large nonstick frying pan or wok over high heat. Add the bacon and spring onions and steam-fry until the onions are soft, adding very small amounts of water as needed to prevent sticking and burning. Add the sprouts and stock and stir-fry for about 3 minutes. Season with the salt and pepper and drizzle with the lemon juice. Toss and serve immediately.

MAKES 8 SERVINGS

Per serving: 71 calories/297 kJ, 12 g protein, 5 g carbohydrates, 1 g sugar, 0.5 g total fat, 6% calories from fat, 2 g fibre, 331 mg sodium

Bulgur Wheat and Quinoa Pilaf

This is a tasty side dish for any meal.

150 g (5½ oz) bulgur wheat
170 g (6 oz) quinoa
1 large onion, chopped
100 g (3½ oz) celery, chopped
1 litre (1¾ pt) low-sodium vegetarian stock
4 tablespoons fresh parsley, finely chopped
1 teaspoon crushed dried rosemary or dried thyme or oregano
Salt to taste

Place the bulgur and quinoa in a dry heavy frying pan (such as cast-iron) or wok over high heat and cook, stirring constantly, until the grain smells toasty. Remove from the heat immediately and set aside.

Steam-fry the onion and celery in a large nonstick saucepan with a tight lid until the onion begins to soften. Add the stock, bulgur, quinoa, parsley and rosemary, thyme or oregano. Bring to the boil over high heat, then reduce the heat to low and cook, covered, for 20 minutes. Let stand for 5 minutes. Fluff with a fork and season with the salt.

MAKES 8 SERVINGS

Per serving: 174 calories/728 kJ, 6 g protein, 36 g carbohydrates, 1 g sugar, 2 g total fat, 7% calories from fat, 6 g fibre, 46 mg sodium

Broccoli Stir-Fry in Black Bean Sauce

This is a colourful, quick and fibre-rich accompaniment to any Oriental-style meal.

1 teaspoon finely chopped or grated fresh ginger
2 teaspoons crushed garlic
2 tablespoons Chinese black bean sauce
1 bunch broccoli
1 large onion, cut into 6 wedges and layers separated
2 tablespoons water
3 tablespoons dry sherry or sweet wine, such as Riesling
1½ teaspoons cornflour dissolved in 120 ml (4 fl oz) cold water

Mash the ginger and garlic together in a small bowl. Add the black bean sauce and mix well.

Divide the broccoli florets into bite-size pieces. Peel and chop the stems into 1 cm (½ in) pieces and stir-fry with the florets and onion in a medium frying pan over high heat. Add 2 tablespoons water, cover and cook for 4 to 5 minutes or just until the broccoli is crisp-tender (add a little more water if necessary).

Add the ginger mixture, sherry or wine, and cornflour mixture and stir until the sauce is thickened. Serve immediately.

MAKES 4 SERVINGS

Per serving: 85 calories/356 kJ, 6 g protein, 15 g carbohydrates, 1 g sugar, 1 g total fat, 4% calories from fat, 0.5 g fibre, 416 mg sodium

Roasted Sweet Potatoes with Moroccan Spices

These sweet potatoes are easy to prepare, but your guests don't have to know that. The seeds add crunch as well as spice.

685 g (1½ lb) orange-fleshed sweet potatoes, peeled, halved
    lengthwise and cut crosswise into 1 cm (½ in) slices
60 ml (2 fl oz) fat-free Italian dressing
1 tablespoon maple syrup
1½ teaspoons grated lemon peel
1½ teaspoons coriander seeds
1½ teaspoons cumin seeds
1½ teaspoons mustard seeds
Salt to taste
Freshly ground black pepper to taste

Position a rack in the bottom third of the oven and preheat the oven to 190°C/375°F/gas 5.

Toss the sweet potatoes, dressing, maple syrup, lemon peel and coriander, cumin and mustard seeds together in a heavy nonstick rimmed baking sheet or shallow baking tray, then spread evenly in a shallow layer. Sprinkle with salt and pepper. Roast until tender and golden brown, stirring occasionally, for 30 to 45 minutes. Serve hot.

MAKES 5 SERVINGS

Per serving: 145 calories/607 kJ, 3 g protein, 33 g carbohydrates, 9 g sugar, 1 g total fat, 3% calories from fat, 5 g fibre, 233 mg sodium

Roasted Green Beans, Fennel, Red Pepper and Cauliflower with Dill

This is a delicious, easy and colourful vegetable presentation.

2 medium fennel bulbs, tops cut off, halved, trimmed and sliced
1 medium cauliflower, trimmed, broken into florets and sliced
2 large red peppers, cored, seeded and thickly sliced
650 g (1 lb 7 oz) fresh green beans, trimmed, or frozen whole
   young green beans
120 ml (4 fl oz) fat-free Italian dressing
2 tablespoons lemon juice
2 teaspoons dried dill weed or 2 tablespoons chopped fresh dill
1 teaspoon dried garlic granules
Salt to taste
Freshly ground black pepper to taste

Preheat the oven to 180°C/350°F/gas 4. Combine the fennel, cauliflower, peppers, beans, dressing, lemon juice, dill, garlic granules, salt and black pepper in a single layer in a large, shallow nonstick baking tray (use two if necessary to keep the vegetables in 1 shallow layer).

Place the tray or trays on the bottom oven rack. Bake for about 40 minutes, stirring occasionally with a spatula, until the vegetables are tender and beginning to brown slightly. Serve hot.

MAKES 8 SERVINGS

Per serving: 85 calories/356 kJ, 4 g protein, 19 g carbohydrates, 6 g sugar, 0.5 g total fat, 3% calories from fat, 7 g fibre, 254 mg sodium

Desserts and Sweet Treats

Gingerbread Cakes

Use a food processor or blender to whip up these spicy treats. They're delicious with apple butter or low-sugar apricot jam. For a special treat, fill them with Lemon Crème (page 242). As with all fat-free baked goods, eat them the day they are made, or freeze, well-wrapped, for future use.

230 g (8 oz) reduced-fat extra-firm silken tofu
170 g (6 oz) molasses (dark or light, according to your taste)
60 g (2 oz) soft brown sugar
6 tablespoons water
170 g (6 oz) wholemeal flour
6 tablespoons barley flour
1 tablespoon ground ginger
1 teaspoon bicarbonate of soda
1 teaspoon baking powder
1 teaspoon ground cinnamon
½ teaspoon salt
¼ teaspoon ground allspice

Preheat the oven to 160°C/325°F/gas 3.

Combine the tofu, molasses, brown sugar and water in a blender or food processor, or with a hand blender, until smooth.

Whisk the wholemeal flour, barley flour, ginger, bicarbonate of soda, baking powder, cinnamon, salt and allspice together well in a medium bowl. Pour in the tofu mixture and mix briefly. Spoon the batter evenly into a nonstick 12-cup muffin tray. Bake for 20 to 25 minutes. Remove the cakes carefully from the tray and cool on a rack, covered with a clean tea towel.

MAKES 12 SERVINGS

Per cupcake: 133 calories/557 kJ, 4 g protein, 28 g carbohydrates, 5 g sugar, 1 g total fat, 8% calories from fat, 3 g fibre, 196 mg sodium

Orange and Apple Date Cake

This easy lunchbox cake is moist and delicious – and even better the next day. The apple sauce replaces both eggs and fat. If you have trouble finding unsweetened apple sauce in your local supermarket, try the baby foods section – or make your own by simmering chopped sweet apples in a little water until soft.

240 ml (8 fl oz) unsweetened smooth apple sauce
1 tablespoon lemon juice
2 tablespoons water
1 tablespoon grated orange peel
145 g (5 oz) wholemeal flour
90 g (3 oz) brown sugar
40 g (1¼ oz) oat flour or barley flour
½ teaspoon ground cinnamon
¼ teaspoon salt
⅛ teaspoon ground nutmeg
⅛ teaspoon ground allspice
1 teaspoon bicarbonate of soda
180 g (6½ oz) chopped pitted dates

Preheat the oven to 180°C/350°F/gas 4. Place the apple sauce, lemon juice and 2 tablespoons water in a small saucepan over medium heat and warm slowly. Add the orange peel.

Mix the flour, brown sugar, oat or barley flour, cinnamon, salt, nutmeg and allspice in a medium bowl.

Stir the bicarbonate of soda into the apple sauce mixture (it will foam up). Pour immediately into the flour mixture and stir briefly but thoroughly.

Add the dates and mix briefly. Scoop the batter into a nonstick 23 cm (9 in) cake tin, smooth the top and bake for 10 minutes. Reduce the heat to 160°C/325°F/gas 3 and bake for 25 to 30 minutes or until firm to the touch. Transfer to a rack and cool completely. Make 2 evenly spaced cuts through the cake vertically, then horizontally, to make 9 squares.

MAKES 9 SERVINGS

Per serving: 169 calories/707 kJ, 3 g protein, 41 g carbohydrates, 24 g sugar, 0.5 g total fat, 2% calories from fat, 4 g fibre, 199 mg sodium

Lemon Crème

This simply delicious crème can be used as a pudding or a topping for fruit or cake. All you need are three ingredients.

340 g (12 oz) reduced-fat extra-firm silken tofu, crumbled
80 ml (3 fl oz) light maple syrup or agave nectar
3 tablespoons fresh lemon juice
1 tablespoon grated lemon peel

Blend the tofu, maple syrup or agave nectar, lemon juice and lemon peel until very smooth in a blender or food processor (or place in a bowl and use a hand-held blender). Refrigerate in a covered container until chilled.

MAKES 4 SERVINGS

Per serving: 106 calories/444 kJ, 6 g protein, 20 g carbohydrates, 17 g sugar, 1 g total fat, 5% calories from fat, 0.5 g fibre, 88 mg sodium

Crispy Fruit Chimichangas

This baked version of a deep-fried Mexican snack food makes a delicious and easy dessert. You can multiply it as needed.

170 g (6 oz) chopped fresh peaches or nectarines
1 wholewheat tortilla
1 tablespoon reduced-fat soya milk
1 teaspoon cinnamon sugar
2 tablespoons Lemon Crème (see above)

Preheat the oven to 260°C/500°F/highest gas setting. Place the fruit in the lower-middle of the tortilla. Fold up the bottom, then fold in the sides, and roll up (like a burrito).

Brush the tortilla all over with some of the soya milk. Place seam-side-down on a nonstick baking sheet, or a baking sheet lined with cooking parchment. Bake for 8 to 10 minutes, or until golden brown and crispy, brushing once or twice again with the remaining soya milk.

To serve, sprinkle with the cinnamon sugar and drizzle the Lemon Crème over the top.

MAKES 2 SERVINGS

Per ½ tortilla: 135 calories/565 kJ, 5 g protein, 27 g carbohydrates, 14 g sugar, 2 g total fat, 12% calories from fat, 2 g fibre, 211 mg sodium

Pineapple Lolly Pops

You can make this variation on a favourite summer treat with a blender and just six ingredients.

340 g (12 oz) reduced-fat firm or extra-firm silken tofu
3 tablespoons agave nectar or 60 g (2 oz) sugar
4 teaspoons lemon juice
¾ teaspoon vanilla extract
400 g (14 oz) juice-packed unsweetened crushed pineapple
¼ teaspoon coconut extract

Place the tofu, agave nectar or sugar, lemon juice, vanilla extract, pineapple (with juice) and coconut extract in a blender and process until smooth. Pour into 18 small lolly pop moulds, insert sticks and freeze until solid. To serve, dip the bottoms of the moulds in hot water for a few seconds so the lollies slide out easily.

MAKES 18 SERVINGS

Per lolly pop: 30 calories/126 kJ, 2 g protein, 6 g carbohydrates, 6 g sugar, 0.5 g total fat, 4% calories from fat, 0.5 g fibre, 19 mg sodium

Berry Mousse

This is so easy that it's hardly a recipe! Your blender does most of the work. This can be eaten as a pudding or used as a topping for fruit.

340 g (12 oz) reduced-fat extra-firm silken tofu, crumbled
340 g (12 oz) frozen unsweetened berries of choice, thawed
3 tablespoons sugar or 2 tablespoons agave nectar
1 tablespoon berry liqueur (optional)

Blend the tofu, berries, sugar or agave nectar and liqueur, if desired, in a blender or food processor until smooth. Spoon into 4 pudding dishes and refrigerate until chilled.

MAKES 4 SERVINGS

Per serving: 123 calories/515 kJ, 7 g protein, 24 g carbohydrates, 17 g sugar, 1 g total fat, 5% calories from fat, 3 g fibre, 89 mg sodium

APPENDIX 1
DIABETES MEDICATIONS

Let's take a look at the medications doctors often prescribe for diabetes. Whether your goal is to get off your medications altogether or to be on as little as possible, you will want to understand what you are taking and why.

Some diabetes medications make it easier to lose weight, but most make it harder. Also, as you will see, when your body is regaining health, doses of some medications need to be trimmed back faster than others.

INSULIN

Insulin is available in a variety of forms that differ mainly in how long they work. Fast-acting insulin lasts for 4 to 6 hours, and regular insulin lasts 5 to 8 hours. Other forms, such as NPH, lente and ultralente, last longer.

Insulin glargine (Lantus) and insulin detemir (Levemir) last a whole day, more or less, and stay at a fairly constant level in the blood, unlike other forms, whose action rises and falls more sharply. Sometimes doctors prescribe long-acting insulin, to be sure that some insulin is in your blood at all times, along with doses of shorter-acting insulin at mealtimes. Insulin is also available in premixed combinations of long-acting and short-acting forms, such as 70/30 (typically, 70 per cent NPH insulin and 30 per cent regular insulin).

Insulin may be administered by injection using syringes; prefilled, multiuse disposable pens; or disposable, multiuse cartridges that are placed into a reusable penlike device. Insulin may also be administered with an insulin pump.

In 2006, a type of fast-acting inhalable insulin was approved for use in adults. Sold under the name Exubera, its long-term safety remains unclear, particularly since it appears to reduce the amount of air the lungs can hold.

Insulin is essential for people with type 1 diabetes and also is used by many with type 2. Unfortunately, most types of insulin make weight loss more difficult, and all types can cause blood sugar to drop too low if you take too much or are not eating enough food.

An additional injectable medication can be used with insulin to improve its action.

ORAL MEDICATIONS

When diet changes do not adequately control type 2 diabetes, doctors typically add oral medications. Commonly used drugs are listed below, with brand names in parentheses.

Metformin (Glucophage) decreases the liver's production of glucose and sensitizes the body to insulin's action. Digestive upset is a common side effect, but it typically disappears with continued use. Metformin does not contribute to weight gain and, when taken by itself, does not cause low blood sugar.

Glipizide (Glibenese, Minodiab), **glimepiride** (Amaryl) and **gliclazide** (Diamicron) are collectively referred to as sulfonylureas. They stimulate the pancreas to release more insulin and are usually taken before meals. Like insulin, they can cause weight gain and can cause blood sugar to drop too low if your food intake does not keep up with the medication. They are the least expensive oral medications but often lose their efficacy after several years of use.

Nateglinide (Starlix) and **repaglinide** (Novonorm) stimulate your pancreas to release insulin for a few hours. They can cause blood sugar to drop too low, although they are less likely to do so than insulin and the sulfonylureas. They must be taken before each meal to be effective.

Pioglitazone (Actos) and **rosiglitazone** (Avandia) increase insulin sensitivity and decrease the liver's production of glucose. They are in the chemical category called thiazolidinediones. They can cause weight gain and fluid retention, but when taken alone, they do not cause low blood sugar.

Acarbose (Glucobay) blocks the enzymes that digest carbohydrate in the intestinal tract and reduce the body's absorption of glucose. Wind and diarrhoea are common side effects.

APPENDIX 2
INGREDIENTS THAT MAY BE NEW TO YOU

The recipes in this book use simple ingredients that are widely available, but a few include ingredients that may be unfamiliar. If you cannot find them at your favourite stores, see Appendix 3 for some convenient online sources.

AGAVE NECTAR

Agave nectar (or syrup) is a mild-flavoured liquid sweetener made from the blue agave cactus plant. Because its sugars are about 90 per cent fructose, which is sweeter than table sugar, you will need to use only about half as much of it as you would sugar. It is available online and in health food stores.

BREADCRUMBS

To make your own, start with leftover sprouted-grain bread, stone-ground wholemeal bread or rye bread that you have torn and saved in a bag in the freezer. When you are ready to make breadcrumbs, just grind the bread pieces in a food processor. Store them in a bag or plastic container in the freezer.

For toasted breadcrumbs, cook in a dry heavy frying pan over medium heat, stirring often and watching constantly, until golden. Let cool thoroughly and store in a covered container.

For dried breadcrumbs, save the bread in a paper bag until hard and dry, then grind. When the crumbs are very dry, they will keep indefinitely in a dry, covered container.

For cheesy breadcrumbs, which are excellent for breading oven-fried vegetables, mix 455 g (1 lb) fine fresh breadcrumbs with 75 g (2½ oz) vegan Parmesan, 1½ teaspoons salt and ½ teaspoon freshly ground black pepper. Keep frozen.

For seasoned breadcrumbs, add the following to plain or cheesy breadcrumbs: 2 tablespoons dried parsley, 1½ tablespoons dried oregano, ½ tablespoon dried basil and ¼ teaspoon dried garlic granules.

CHICKPEA FLOUR (BESAN)

This flour, ground dried chickpeas, makes a good substitute for soya flour. It is similar in fat content to low-fat soya flour and is high in fibre and protein. It is available in health food stores and some large supermarkets.

FLAXSEED

These small brown or golden seeds are a great source of fibre and omega-3 fatty acids. They must be ground to be digestible. Ground flaxseed is sold refrigerated, or you can buy whole flaxseed and grind a little at a time in a spice mill or coffee grinder to add to shakes, cereals, breadcrumb toppings, baked goods, etc. Most supermarkets and health food stores stock flaxseed.

MEAT SUBSTITUTES

Health food stores and supermarkets now sell a range of vegetarian burgers, sausages, hot dogs, cold meats, meatballs, bacon and 'meat' pieces for stir-fries and casseroles. Most are made from soya or wheat gluten (seitan).

Precooked and ready to eat, they are the ultimate in convenience. Brands vary widely in fat content and ingredients (e.g., some contain egg or dairy products), so check the labels. Health food stores do tend to have a wider range and more products that are vegan.

MISO

Miso is Japanese fermented soyabean and grain paste, usually made with rice or barley. It is a versatile soup base, similar to bouillon paste or cubes, and a savoury flavouring. For those with soya allergies, chickpea miso is available.

MUSHROOM STOCK CUBES

These stock cubes make a rich, savoury stock. They are not widely available in supermarkets but you can find them in some health food stores and on the Internet – often on sites specialising in Italian ingredients.

NUTRITIONAL YEAST

Nutritional yeast adds a cheesy flavour to sauces, casseroles, stir-fries and other dishes. It is not the same as brewer's yeast or baker's yeast, both of which have a bitter flavour. It comes as flakes and powder, and you will find that the flakes are more versatile. You can find it in health food stores. If you can find only the powdered form, use half as much as the amount of flakes called for, since it is more concentrated.

SOYA FLOUR

Soya flour is made from whole or hulled soyabeans. It contains an enzyme, lipoxygenase, that serves as a dough conditioner, producing moist, light bread that tends to stay fresh. Because of its high oil content, soya flour should be kept in the freezer. Defatted varieties are also available.

SOYA MILK AND OTHER NONDAIRY MILKS

Soya milk is available in most supermarkets and health food stores. It can replace cow's milk in cooking as well as on cereal, in hot beverages, etc. It is lactose free, cholesterol free and often fortified with calcium, vitamin D and other nutrients. In recipes, reduced-fat plain soya milk works well. Most brands are lightly sweetened to taste similar to dairy milk, but unsweetened versions may be used in savoury cooking. To avoid curdling in hot beverages, add hot coffee or tea to the soya milk rather than the other way around.

Soya milk should not be used in place of infant formula. Soya-based infant formulas are specifically formulated for babies' needs.

In addition to soya milk, rice milk, oat milk, almond milk and other dairy-free milks are available. All are free of animal fat, animal protein and lactose. Some people prefer them to soya milk.

SOYA CHEESES

Soya cheeses, available at health food stores, are made from tofu and, refrigerated, keep for months. However, many are too high in fat to be suitable, so check the label.

SOYA PROTEIN POWDER (SOYA PROTEIN ISOLATE)

Protein powders are made by removing the fat, fibre and carbohydrates from soyabeans. What remains is mostly protein, with some residual minerals and a trace of fat. The powder is bland, highly digestible and easy to add to shakes and other recipes. It can be used as an emulsifier, binding fat and water together and lending a creamy texture. Plain or flavoured versions are available in health food stores. The powder keeps well without refrigeration.

SOY SAUCE (LOW-SODIUM)

Soy sauce, which originated in China, is one of the oldest condiments in the world. Its rich flavour adds body to many Western meatless recipes. Low-sodium varieties (e.g., Kikkoman) have a health advantage while maintaining the flavour of the original.

SOYA YOGURT

Soya yogurts are available with live bacterial cultures. They have a pleasant, thick texture and the characteristic tartness. While most large supermarkets will stock one brand, you will find more choice in health food stores.

TEXTURED VEGETABLE PROTEIN (TVP)

This useful low-fat product is made by mixing defatted soya flour with water, cooking it at high pressure and extruding the cooked mixture through a machine that makes a variety of textured and shaped products. The result is a versatile product with a surprisingly meaty texture. In granular form (often called soya mince), it replaces ground meat. In chunk form, it works well for stews, kebabs and stir-fries. Cutlets are also available. These products are not widely available in supermarkets, but health food stores will usually stock various forms of TVP.

TVP is easily rehydrated for use in soups, stews, casseroles and sauces. In fact, if your dish is too watery, you can add the vegetable protein in its dry state, and it will absorb the liquid – and its flavour.

To quickly rehydrate granules, mix them with an almost equal amount of very hot or boiling liquid, cover and let stand for 5 minutes. Plain water is fine if the granules will be added to a spicy mixture. If you prefer, you can use stock or tomato juice or just add 1 or 2 table-spoons of low-sodium soy sauce to the hot water.

Chunks and cutlets take a little longer to reconstitute but have an amazingly meatlike texture and a mild flavour. Reconstitute them by cooking the dry product in twice its volume of vegetarian stock for 15 to 30 minutes. Cool and store in the cooking liquid. Drain cutlets and pat dry before marinating or coating with flour and oven frying. Aside from their use in stews and stir-fries, chunks be used in kebabs and oven fried. Just coat with seasoned flour or breadcrumbs and bake at 200°C/400°F/gas 6 for about 10 minutes per side.

TOFU

Tofu is made from soya milk that is curdled with mineral salts and then drained and pressed into various textures. It takes on flavours easily and can be used as a substitute for dairy products, meat, poultry, seafood and eggs.

Some brands are sold in aseptic packages that keep for about a year unopened. Silken tofu has a smooth texture and comes in soft, firm and extra-firm varieties, regular and reduced fat. It works well for blended, creamy mixtures, such as puddings, smoothies, sauces, soups and pie fillings, but can also be used for Tofu Scramblers (see page 192) and other dishes. For stir-fries, regular tofu works better than the silken type.

Health food stores and some supermarkets also sell smoked and mar-inated varieties. In small amounts, they can replace meats, poultry and even smoked fish in stir-fries, sautés, casseroles, salads and sandwiches.

APPENDIX 3
RESOURCES

Support and Advocacy

Diabetes UK
www.diabetes.org.uk
Diabetes UK is the largest organization in the UK working for people with diabetes. It
provides general health advice for diabetics as well as advice on diet.

Diabetes Australia
www.diabetesaustralia.com.au
Diabetes Australia offers personalized and practical assistance for people with diabetes
and their carers.

Diabetes New Zealand
www.diabetes.org.nz
This organization aims to help both sufferers and health professionals. It has a useful
'dear dietitian' tool, where visitors can put their questions to a registered dietitian.

Diabetes South Africa
www.diabetessa.co.za
Diabetes South Africa provides information and advice for people with diabetes and
lobbies for better services and cheaper medications for sufferers.

The International Diabetes Federation
www.idf.org
The IDF is a worldwide alliance of diabetes associations. Its aim is to raise global
awareness of diabetes, promote appropriate diabetes care and prevention, and
encourage research towards finding a cure. It is a good source of information on
what is happening on a worldwide scale.

American Diabetes Association
www.diabetes.org
This comprehensive, user-friendly site is a good source of news, background
information and recipes.

Diabetes Research and Wellness Foundation
www.drwf.org.uk
Established to help people with diabetes and to raise awareness about the disease and its
associated complications, the DRWF also funds research projects. The website is a
useful source of information on ongoing and recent research.

To find a registered dietitian, working in private practice in your area, contact the
British Dietic Association, *www.bda.uk.com.*

Food and Ingredients

For information on the glycaemic index, visit *www.glycemicindex.com*, a service of the University of Sydney, Australia.

The Vegan Society
www.vegansociety.com
This is a good source of advice on replacing animal products in your diet.

Vegan Village
www.veganvillage.co.uk
This website has a wide range of vegan recipes, as well as listings of vegan cafes, restaurants and guesthouses in the UK.

Goodness Direct
www.goodnessdirect.co.uk
This online store sells a wide range of products, including agave nectar, TVP and nutritional yeast.

The Vegan Store
www.veganstore.co.uk
As well as 'cruelty-free' products this site has a range of useful store-cupboard items, including seitan, egg replacer and vegan gelatine.

The Vegetarian Society of Australia
www.vegetariansociety.org.au
This website provides good links to vegan food suppliers and sources of recipes.

Porphry's People
www.vegan.org.nz
The website of this vegan group, who are based in Christchurch, has some good nutritional information and articles.

The South African Vegan Society
www.vegansociety.co.za
A useful site that includes a shopping guide, plus interesting blogs and links.

HappyCow
www.happycow.net
Provides the locations of vegetarian restaurants anywhere in the world. Because restaurants often change, call before you go.

NOTES

INTRODUCTION

[1] World Health Organization, www.who.int/diabetes/facts/world_figures/en/index.html; accessed December 7, 2005.

[2] A. S. Nicholson et al., 'Toward Improved Management of NIDDM: A Randomized, Controlled, Pilot Intervention Using a Low-Fat, Vegetarian Diet', *Preventive Medicine* 29 (1999): 87–91.

[3] N. D. Barnard et al., 'The Effects of a Low-Fat, Plant-Based Dietary Intervention on Body Weight, Metabolism, and Insulin Sensitivity', *American Journal of Medicine* 118 (2005): 991–7.

CHAPTER 1

[1] M. Knip et al., 'Environmental Triggers and Determinants of Type 1 Diabetes', *Diabetes* 54, suppl 2 (December 2005): S125–36.

[2] J. H. Laitinen et al., 'Impact of Intensified Dietary Therapy on Energy and Nutrient Intakes and Fatty Acid Composition of Serum Lipids in Patients with Recently Diagnosed Non-Insulin-Dependent Diabetes Mellitus', *Journal of the American Dietetic Association* 93 (1993): 276–83.

[3] M. J. Franz, P. L. Splett, and A. Monk, 'Cost-Effectiveness of Medical Nutrition Therapy Provided by Dietitians for Persons with Non-Insulin-Dependent Diabetes Mellitus', *Journal of the American Dietetic Association* 95 (1995): 1018–24.

[4] J. B. Buse, C. J. Rubin, and R. Frederich, 'Muraglitazar, a Dual (Alpha/Gamma) PPAR Activator: A Randomized, Double-Blind, Placebo-Controlled, 24-Week Monotherapy Trial in Adult Patients with Type 2 Diabetes', *Clinical Therapeutics* 27 (2005): 1181–95.

[5] Laitinen et al., 'Impact of Intensified Dietary Therapy'.

CHAPTER 2

[1] T. Kuzuya, 'Prevalence of Diabetes Mellitus in Japan Compiled from Literature', *Diabetes Research and Clinical Practice* 24, suppl (1994): S15–21.

[2] H. P. Himsworth, 'The Dietetic Factor Determining the Glucose Tolerance and Sensitivity to Insulin of Healthy Men', *Clinical Science* 2 (1935): 67–94.

[3] D. B. Stone and W. E. Connor, 'The Prolonged Effects of a Low-Cholesterol, High-Carbohydrate Diet upon the Serum Lipids in Diabetic Patients', *Diabetes* 12 (1963): 127–32.

[4] J. W. Anderson and K. Ward, 'High-Carbohydrate, High-Fiber Diets for Insulin-Treated Men with Diabetes Mellitus', *American Journal of Clinical Nutrition* 32 (1979): 2312–21.

[5] R. J. Barnard, T. Jung, and S. B. Inkeles, 'Diet and Exercise in the Treatment of NIDDM: The Need for Early Emphasis', *Diabetes Care* 17 (1994): 1469–72.

[6] A. S. Nicholson et al., 'Toward Improved Management of NIDDM: A Randomized, Controlled, Pilot Intervention Using a Low-Fat, Vegetarian Diet', *Preventive Medicine* 29 (1999): 87–91.

[7] N. D. Barnard et al., 'The Effects of a Low-Fat, Plant-Based Dietary Intervention on Body Weight, Metabolism, and Insulin Sensitivity', *American Journal of Medicine* 118 (2005): 991–7.

[8] Ibid.

[9] UK Prospective Diabetes Study (UKPDS) Group, 'Effect of Intensive Blood-Glucose Control with Metformin on Complications in Overweight Patients with Type 2 Diabetes (UKPDS 34)', *Lancet* 352 (1998): 854–65.

[10] I. M. Stratton, A. L. Adler, and H. A. Neil, 'Association of Glycaemia with Macrovascular and Microvascular Complications of Type 2 Diabetes (UKPDS 35): Prospective Observational Study', *British Medical Journal* 321 (2000): 405–12.

[11] UK Prospective Diabetes Study (UKPDS) Group, 'Effect of Intensive Blood-Glucose Control'.

[12] D. Ornish et al., 'Can Lifestyle Changes Reverse Coronary Heart Disease?' *Lancet* 336 (1990): 129–33.

[13] D. Ornish et al., 'Intensive Lifestyle Changes for Reversal of Coronary Heart Disease', *Journal of the American Medical Association* 280 (1998): 2001–7.

[14] S. Berkow and N. D. Barnard, 'Blood Pressure Regulation and Vegetarian Diets', *Nutrition Reviews* 63 (2005): 1–8.

[15] K. F. Petersen et al., 'Impaired Mitochondrial Activity in the Insulin-Resistant Offspring of Patients with Type 2 Diabetes', *New England Journal of Medicine* 350 (2004): 664–71.

[16] Ibid.

[17] L. M. Sparks et al., 'A High-Fat Diet Coordinately Downregulates Genes Required for Mitochondrial Oxidative Phosphorylation in Skeletal Muscle', *Diabetes* 54 (2005): 1926–33.

[18] A. V. Greco et al, 'Insulin Resistance in Morbid Obesity: Reversal with Intramyocellular Fat Depletion', *Diabetes* 52 (2002): 144–51.

[19] L. M. Goff et al., 'Veganism and Its Relationship with Insulin Resistance and Intramyocellular Lipid', *European Journal of Clinical Nutrition* 59 (2005): 291–8.

CHAPTER 3

[1] D. M. Nathan et al. and the Diabetes Control and Complications Trial/Epidemiology of Diabetes Interventions and Complications (DCCT/EDIC) Study Research Group, 'Intensive Diabetes Treatment and Cardiovascular Disease in Patients with Type 1 Diabetes', *New England Journal of Medicine* 353 (2005): 2643–53.

[2] Diabetes Control and Complications Trial Research Group, 'The Effect of Intensive Treatment of Diabetes on the Development and Progression of Long-Term Complications in Insulin-Dependent Diabetes Mellitus', *New England Journal of Medicine* 329 (1993): 977–86.

[3] E. L. Knight et al., 'The Impact of Protein Intake on Renal Function Decline in Women with Normal Renal Function or Mild Renal Insufficiency', *Annals of Internal Medicine* 138 (2003): 460–7.

[4] J. Karjalainen et al., 'A Bovine Albumin Peptide as a Possible Trigger of Insulin-Dependent Diabetes Mellitus', *New England Journal of Medicine* 327 (1992): 302–7.

[5] A. C. Alting, R. G. J. M. Meijer, and E. C. H. van Beresteijn, 'Incomplete Elimination of the ABBOS Epitope of Bovine Serum Albumin under Simulated Gastrointestinal Conditions of Infants', *Diabetes Care* 20 (1997): 875–80.

[6] D. Hammond-McKibben and H. M. Dosch, 'Cow's Milk, Bovine Serum Albumin, and IDDM: Can We Settle the Controversies?' *Diabetes Care* 20 (1997): 897–901.

[7] Ibid.

[8] American Academy of Pediatrics Work Group on Cow's Milk Protein and Diabetes Mellitus, 'Infant Feeding Practices and Their Possible Relationship to the Etiology of Diabetes Mellitus', *Pediatrics* 94 (1994): 752–4.

[9] H. K. Akerblom et al., 'Dietary Manipulation of Beta Cell Autoimmunity in Infants at Increased Risk of Type 1 Diabetes: A Pilot Study', *Diabetologia* 48 (2005): 829–37.

[10] P. S. Clyne and A. Kulczycki Jr., 'Human Breast Milk Contains Bovine IgG: Relationship to Infant Colic?' *Pediatrics* 87 (1991): 439–44.

[11] K. Sadeharju et al., 'Enterovirus Infections as a Risk Factor for Type 1 Diabetes: Virus Analyses in a Dietary Intervention Trial', *Clinical and Experimental Immunology* 132 (2003): 271–7.

CHAPTER 4

1   L. M. Goff et al., 'Veganism and Its Relationship with Insulin Resistance and Intramyocellular Lipid', *European Journal of Clinical Nutrition* 59 (2005): 291–8.

2   L. Hooper et al., 'Risks and Benefits of Omega 3 Fats for Mortality, Cardiovascular Disease, and Cancer: Systematic Review', *British Medical Journal* 332 (2006): 752–60.

3   D. B. Hunninghake et al., 'The Efficacy of Intensive Dietary Therapy Alone or Combined with Lovastatin in Outpatients with Hypercholesterolemia', *New England Journal of Medicine* 328 (1993): 1213–19.

4   E. L. Knight et al., 'The Impact of Protein Intake on Renal Function Decline in Women with Normal Renal Function or Mild Renal Insufficiency', *Annals of Internal Medicine* 138 (2003): 460–7.

5   E. Giovannucci et al., 'Calcium and Fructose Intake in Relation to Risk of Prostate Cancer', *Cancer Research* 58 (1998): 442–7.

6   J. M. Chan et al., 'Dairy Products, Calcium, and Prostate Cancer Risk in the Physicians' Health Study', *American Journal of Clinical Nutrition* 74 (2001): 549–54.

7   S. C. Larsson, N. Orsini, and A. Wolk, 'Milk, Milk Products and Lactose Intake and Ovarian Cancer Risk: A Meta-Analysis of Epidemiological Studies', *International Journal of Cancer* 118 (2006): 431–41.

8   J. M. Genkinger et al., 'Dairy Products and Ovarian Cancer: A Pooled Analysis of 12 Cohort Studies', *Cancer Epidemiology Biomarkers & Prevention* 15 (2006): 364–72.

9   D. J. Jenkins et al., 'Glycemic Index of Foods: A Physiological Basis for Carbohydrate Exchange', *American Journal of Clinical Nutrition* 34 (1981): 362–6.

10 Ibid.

11 J. Brand-Miller et al., 'Low-Glycemic Index Diets in the Management of Diabetes', *Diabetes Care* 26 (2003): 2261–7.

12 N. C. Howarth, E. Saltzman, and S. B. Roberts, 'Dietary Fiber and Weight Regulation', *Nutrition Reviews* 59 (2001): 129–39.

13 N. D. Barnard et al., 'The Effects of a Low-Fat, Plant-Based Dietary Intervention on Body Weight, Metabolism, and Insulin Sensitivity', *American Journal of Medicine* 118 (2005): 991–7.

14 M. G. Crane and C. Sample, 'Regression of Diabetic Neuropathy with Total Vegetarian (Vegan) Diet', *Journal of Nutritional Medicine* 4 (1994): 431–9.

15 Y. Papanikolaou et al., 'Bean Consumption by Adults Is Associated with a More Nutrient Dense Diet and a Reduced Risk of Obesity', presented at the Experimental Biology Conference, April 1–5, 2006, San Francisco, CA.

16 V. L. Fulgoni et al., 'Bean Consumption by Children Is Associated with Better Nutrient Intake and Lower Body Weights and Waist Circumferences', presented at the Experimental Biology Conference, April 1–5, 2006, San Francisco, CA.

17 J. W. Anderson and A. W. Major, 'Pulses and Lipaemia, Short- and Long-Term Effect: Potential in the Prevention of Cardiovascular Disease', *British Journal of Nutrition* 88, suppl 3 (2002): S263–71.

18 M. Saito et al., 'Undesirable Effects of Citrus Juice on the Pharmacokinetics of Drugs: Focus on Recent Studies', *Drug Safety* 28 (2005): 677–94.

19 G. M. Turner-McGrievy et al., 'Effects of a Low-Fat, Vegan Diet and a Step II Diet on Macro- and Micronutrient Intakes in Overweight, Postmenopausal Women', *Nutrition* 20 (2004): 738–46.

20 Knight et al., 'The Impact of Protein Intake'.

21 American Dietetic Association, 'Position of the American Dietetic Association and Dietitians of Canada: Vegetarian Diets', *Journal of the American Dietetic Association* 103 (2003): 748–65.

22 D. Feskanich, W. C. Willett, and G. A. Colditz, 'Calcium, Vitamin D, Milk Consumption, and Hip Fractures: A Prospective Study among Postmenopausal Women', *American Journal of Clinical Nutrition* 77 (2003): 504–11.

[23] E. C. Westman et al., 'Effect of a 6-Month Adherence to a Very Low Carbohydrate Diet Program', *American Journal of Medicine* 113 (2002): 30–6.

CHAPTER 6

[1] E. L. Knight et al., 'The Impact of Protein Intake on Renal Function Decline in Women with Normal Renal Function or Mild Renal Insufficiency', *Annals of Internal Medicine* 138 (2003): 460–7.

[2] J. Coresh et al., 'Prevalence of Chronic Kidney Disease and Decreased Kidney Function in the Adult US Population: Third National Health and Nutrition Examination Survey', *American Journal of Kidney Diseases* 41 (2003): 1–12.

[3] A. M. Dattilo and P. M. Kris-Etherton, 'Effects of Weight Reduction on Blood Lipids and Lipoproteins: A Meta-Analysis', *American Journal of Clinical Nutrition* 56 (1992): 320–8.

[4] E. C. Westman et al., 'Effect of a 6-Month Adherence to a Very Low Carbohydrate Diet Program', *American Journal of Medicine* 113 (2002): 30–6.

[5] W. S. Yancy et al., 'A Low-Carbohydrate, Ketogenic Diet versus a Low-Fat Diet to Treat Obesity and Hyperlipidemia', *Annals of Internal Medicine* 130 (2004): 769–77.

[6] N. D. Barnard et al., 'The Effects of a Low-Fat, Plant-Based Dietary Intervention on Body Weight, Metabolism, and Insulin Sensitivity', *American Journal of Medicine* 118 (2005): 991–7.

[7] A. S. Nicholson et al., 'Toward Improved Management of NIDDM: A Randomized, Controlled, Pilot Intervention Using a Low-Fat, Vegetarian Diet', *Preventive Medicine* 29 (1999): 87–91.

[8] N. C. Howarth, E. Saltzman, and S. B. Roberts, 'Dietary Fiber and Weight Regulation', *Nutrition Reviews* 59 (2001): 129–39.

[9] Barnard et al., 'The Effects of a Low-Fat, Plant-Based Dietary Intervention'.

[10] B. Rolls and R. A. Barnett, *The Volumetrics Weight-Control Plan* (New York: Quill, 2000).

[11] Dattilo and Kris-Etherton, 'Effects of Weight Reduction'.

CHAPTER 7

[1] G. B. Bolli and J. E. Gerich, 'The "Dawn Phenomenon"—A Common Occurrence in Both Non-Insulin-Dependent and Insulin-Dependent Diabetes Mellitus', *New England Journal of Medicine* 310 (1984): 746–50.

[2] E. Selvin et al., 'Meta-analysis: A1c and Cardiovascular Disease in Diabetes Mellitus', *Annals of Internal Medicine* 141 (2004): 421–31.

[3] National Cholesterol Education Program, 'Third Report of the National Cholesterol Education Program (NCEP) Expert Panel on Detection, Evaluation, and Treatment of High Blood Cholesterol in Adults (Adult Treatment Panel III) Final Report', *Circulation* 106 (2002): 3143–421.

[4] American Diabetes Association, 'Standards of Medical Care in Diabetes—2006', *Diabetes Care* 29, suppl 1 (2006): S4–42.

[5] S. M. Grundy et al., 'Implications of Recent Clinical Trials for the National Cholesterol Education Program Adult Treatment Panel III Guidelines', *Circulation* 110 (2004): 227–39.

CHAPTER 9

[1] M. R. Yeomans et al., 'Effects of Nalmefene on Feeding in Humans', *Psychopharmacology* 100 (1990): 426–32.

[2] D. J. Jenkins et al., 'Low-Glycemic Index Diet in Hyperlipidemia: Use of Traditional Starchy Foods', *American Journal of Clinical Nutrition* 46 (1987): 66–71.

[3] Y. Hata and K. Nakajima, 'Life-Style and Serum Lipids and Lipoproteins', *Journal of Atherosclerosois & Thrombosis* 7 (2000): 177–97.

[4] Ibid.

[5] M. J. Malloy and K. P. Kane, 'A Risk Factor for Atherosclerosis: Triglyceride-Rich Lipoproteins', *Advances in Internal Medicine* 47 (2001): 111–36.

CHAPTER 10

[1] R. H. Fletcher and K. M. Fairfield, 'Vitamins for Chronic Disease Prevention in Adults: Clinical Applications', *Journal of the American Medical Association* 287 (2002): 3127–9.

[2] A. Khan et al., 'Cinnamon Improves Glucose and Lipids of People with Type 2 Diabetes', *Diabetes Care* 26 (2003): 3215–18.

[3] R. A. Anderson et al., 'Isolation and Characterization of Polyphenol Type-A Polymers from Cinnamon with Insulin-Like Biological Activity', *Journal of Agricultural & Food Chemistry* 52 (2004): 65–70.

[4] Y. Song et al., 'Dietary Magnesium Intake in Relation to Plasma Insulin Levels and Risk of Type 2 Diabetes in Women', *Diabetes Care* 37(1) (2004): 59–65.

[5] W. Mertz, 'Chromium Occurrence and Function in Biological Systems', *Physiological Reviews* 49 (1969): 163–239.

[6] K. N. Jeejeebhoy et al., 'Chromium Deficiency, Glucose Intolerance, and Neuropathy Reversed by Chromium Supplementation in a Patient Receiving Long-Term Total Parenteral Nutrition', *American Journal of Clinical Nutrition* 30 (1977): 531–8.

[7] N. Kleefstra et al., 'Chromium Treatment Has No Effect in Patients with Poorly Controlled, Insulin-Treated Type 2 Diabetes in an Obese Western Population', *Diabetes Care* 29 (2006): 521–5.

[8] G. J. Ryan et al., 'Chromium as Adjunctive Treatment for Type 2 Diabetes', *American Pharmacy* 37 (2003): 876–85.

[9] W. T. Cefalu and F. B. Hu, 'Role of Chromium in Human Health and in Diabetes', *Diabetes Care* 27 (2004): 2741–51.

[10] S. Jacob et al., 'Oral Administration of RAC-lipoic Acid Modulates Insulin Sensitivity in Patients with Type-2 Diabetes Mellitus: A Placebo-Controlled Pilot Trial', *Free Radical Biology & Medicine* 27 (1999): 309–14.

[11] D. Ziegler, 'Thioctic Acid for Patients with Symptomatic Diabetic Polyneuropathy: A Critical Review', *Treatments in Endocrinology* 3 (2004): 173–89.

CHAPTER 11

[1] W. C. Knowler et al., 'Reduction in the Incidence of Type 2 Diabetes with Lifestyle Intervention or Metformin', *New England Journal of Medicine* 346 (2002): 393–403.

[2] N. G. Boulé et al., 'Effects of Exercise on Glycemic Control and Body Mass in Type 2 Diabetes Mellitus: A Meta-Analysis of Controlled Clinical Trials', *Journal of the American Medical Association* 286 (2001): 1218–27.

[3] C. C. Curioni and P. M. Lourenco, 'Long-Term Weight Loss after Diet and Exercise: A Systematic Review', *International Journal of Obesity (London)* 29 (2005): 1168–74.

[4] Boulé et al., 'Effects of Exercise'.

[5] G. Hu et al., 'Physical Activity, Cardiovascular Risk Factors, and Mortality among Finnish Adults with Diabetes', *Diabetes Care* 28 (2005): 799–805.

[6] G. Hu et al. 'Leisure Time, Occupational, and Commuting Physical Activity and the Risk of Stroke', *Stroke* 36 (2005): 1994–9.

[7] M. J. Tansey and the Diabetes Research in Children Network (DirecNet) Study Group, 'The Effects of Aerobic Exercise on Glucose and Counterregulatory Hormone Concentrations in Children with Type 1 Diabetes', *Diabetes Care* 29 (2006): 20–5.

[8] R. J. Sigal et al., 'Physical Activity/Exercise and Type 2 Diabetes', *Diabetes Care* 27 (2004): 2518–39.

CHAPTER 12

[1] S. Manley, 'Haemoglobin A1c—A Marker for Complications of Type 2 Diabetes: The Experience from the UK Prospective Diabetes Study (UKPDS)', *Clinical Chemistry and Laboratory Medicine* 41 (2003): 1182–90.

[2] E. Selvin et al., 'Meta-Analysis: A1c and Cardiovascular Disease in Diabetes Mellitus', *Annals of Internal Medicine* 141 (2004): 421–31.

[3] D. B. Hunninghake et al., 'The Efficacy of Intensive Dietary Therapy Alone or Combined with Lovastatin in Outpatients with Hypercholesterolemia', *New England Journal of Medicine* 328 (1993): 1213–19.

[4] N. D. Barnard, L. W. Scherwitz, and D. Ornish. 'Adherence and Acceptability of a Low-Fat, Vegetarian Diet among Patients with Cardiac Disease', *Journal of Cardiopulmonary Rehabilitation* 12 (1992): 423–31.

[5] D. Ornish et al., 'Can Lifestyle Changes Reverse Coronary Heart Disease?' *Lancet* 336 (1990): 129–33.

[6] D. Ornish et al., 'Intensive Lifestyle Changes for Reversal of Coronary Heart Disease', *Journal of the American Medical Association* 280 (1998): 2001–7.

[7] N. D. Barnard, A. Akhtar, and A. Nicholson, 'Factors That Facilitate Compliance to Lower Fat Intake', *Archives of Family Medicine* 4 (1995): 153–8.

[8] C. B. Esselstyn Jr., 'Updating a 12-Year Experience with Arrest and Reversal Therapy for Coronary Heart Disease (an Overdue Requiem for Palliative Cardiology)', *American Journal of Cardiology* 84 (1999): 339–41.

[9] J. W. Anderson, B. M. Smith, and C. S. Washnock, 'Cardiovascular and Renal Benefits of Dry Bean and Soybean Intake', *American Journal of Clinical Nutrition* 70, suppl 3 (1999): 464S–74S.

[10] M. Messina and V. Messina, *The Simple Soybean and Your Health* (Garden City Park, NY: Avery, 1994).

[11] E. B. Feldman, 'The Scientific Evidence for a Beneficial Health Relationship between Walnuts and Coronary Heart Disease', *Journal of Nutrition* 132 (2002): 1062S–101S.

[12] R. A. Nagourney, 'Garlic: Medicinal Food or Nutritious Medicine?' *Journal of Medicinal Food* 1 (1998): 13–128.

[13] J. D. Belcher et al., 'Vitamin E, LDL, and Endothelium: Brief Oral Vitamin Supplementation Prevents Oxidized LDL-Mediated Vascular Injury in Vitro', *Arteriosclerosis & Thrombosis* 13 (1993): 1779–89.

[14] D. J. Jenkins et al., 'Direct Comparison of a Dietary Portfolio of Cholesterol-Lowering Foods with a Statin in Hypercholesterolemic Participants', *American Journal of Clinical Nutrition* 81 (2005): 380–7.

[15] A. M. Dattilo and P. M. Kris-Etherton, 'Effects of Weight Reduction on Blood Lipids and Lipoproteins: A Meta-Analysis', *American Journal of Clinical Nutrition* 56 (1992): 320–8.

[16] W. E. Kraus et al., 'Effects of the Amount and Intensity of Exercise on Plasma Lipoproteins', *New England Journal of Medicine* 347 (2002): 1483–92.

[17] D. J. Jenkins et al., 'Low-Glycemic Index Diet in Hyperlipidemia: Use of Traditional Starchy Foods', *American Journal of Clinical Nutrition* 46 (1987): 66–71.

[18] Anderson, Smith, and Washnock, 'Cardiovascular and Renal Benefits'.

[19] Homocysteine Studies Collaboration, 'Homocysteine and Risk of Ischemic Heart Disease and Stroke: A Meta-Analysis', *Journal of the American Medical Association* 288 (2002): 2015–22.

[20] Jenkins et al., 'Low-Glycemic Index Diet'.

[21] S. Berkow and N. D. Barnard, 'Blood Pressure Regulation and Vegetarian Diets', *Nutrition Reviews* 63 (2005): 1–8.

CHAPTER 13

[1] M. G. Crane, 'Sample C. Regression of Diabetic Neuropathy with Total Vegetarian (Vegan) Diet', *Journal of Nutritional Medicine* 4 (1994): 431–9.

[2] D. Ziegler, 'Thioctic Acid for Patients with Symptomatic Diabetic Polyneuropathy: A Critical Review', *Treatments in Endocrinology* 3 (2004): 173–89.

[3] D. F. Horrobin, 'Essential Fatty Acids in the Management of Impaired Nerve Function in Diabetes', *Diabetes* 46, suppl 2 (1997): S90–3.

4 A. A. Sima et al. and the Acetyl-L-Carnitine Study Group, 'Acetyl-L-Carnitine Improves Pain, Nerve Regeneration, and Vibratory Perception in Patients with Chronic Diabetic Neuropathy: An Analysis of Two Randomized Placebo-Controlled Trials', *Diabetes Care* 28 (2005): 89–94.

5 I. De Leeuw et al., 'Long Term Magnesium Supplementation Influences Favourably the Natural Evolution of Neuropathy in Mg-Depleted Type 1 Diabetic Patients (T1dm)', *Magnesium Research* 17 (2004): 109–14.

6 M. Lu et al., 'Prospective Study of Dietary Fat and Risk of Cataract Extraction among US Women', *American Journal of Epidemiology* 161 (2005): 948–59.

7 I. Birlouez-Aragon et al., 'Disturbed Galactose Metabolism in Elderly and Diabetic Humans Is Associated with Cataract Formation', *Journal of Nutrition* 123 (1993): 1370–6.

8 L. Brown et al., 'A Prospective Study of Carotenoid Intake and Risk of Cataract Extraction in US Men', *American Journal of Clinical Nutrition* 70 (1999): 517–24.

9 K. J. Yeum et al., 'Measurement of Carotenoids, Retinoids, and Tocopherols in Human Lenses', *Investigative Ophthalmology & Visual Science* 36 (1995): 2756–61.

10 R. G. Cumming, P. Mitchell, and W. Smith, 'Diet and Cataract: The Blue Mountains Eye Study', *Ophthalmology* 107 (2000): 450–6.

11 M. S. Morris et al., 'Moderate Alcoholic Beverage Intake and Early Nuclear and Cortical Lens Opacities', *Ophthalmic Epidemiology* 11 (2004): 53–65.

12 Y. Ohkubo et al., 'Intensive Insulin Therapy Prevents the Progression of Diabetic Microvascular Complications in Japanese Patients with Non-Insulin-Dependent Diabetes Mellitus: A Randomized Prospective 6-Year Study', *Diabetes Research & Clinical Practice* 28 (1995): 103–17.

13 J. P. Mathews, D. Mathews, and M. J. Lavin, 'The Management of Diabetic Retinopathy', *Practitioner* 248 (2004): 34, 38–42.

14 D. S. Fong et al., Early Treatment Diabetic Retinopathy Study Research Group, 'Causes of Severe Visual Loss in the Early Treatment Diabetic Retinopathy Study: ETDRS Report no. 24', *American Journal of Ophthalmology* 127 (1999): 137–41.

15 K. S. Lam et al., 'Cholesterol-Lowering Therapy May Retard the Progression of Diabetic Nephropathy', *Diabetologia* 38 (1995): 604–9.

16 M. T. Pedrini et al., 'The Effects of Dietary Protein Restriction on the Progression of Diabetic and Non-Diabetic Renal Disease: A Meta-Analysis', *Annals of Internal Medicine* 124 (1996): 627–32.

17 M. M. Jibani et al., 'Predominantly Vegetarian Diet in Patients with Incipient and Early Clinical Diabetic Nephropathy: Effects on Albumin Excretion Rate and Nutritional Status', *Diabetic Medicine* 8 (1991): 949–53.

18 L. Azadbakht et al., 'Beneficiary Effect of Dietary Soy Protein on Lowering Plasma Levels of Lipid and Improving Kidney Function in Type II Diabetes with Nephropathy', *European Journal of Clinical Nutrition* 57 (2003): 1292–4.

19 S. Berkow and N. D. Barnard, 'Blood Pressure Regulation and Vegetarian Diets', *Nutrition Reviews* 63 (2005): 1–8.

INDEX